Why Hospitals Fail

Prasad Godbole • Derek Burke
Jill Aylott
Editors

Why Hospitals Fail

Between Theory and Practice

Springer

Editors
Prasad Godbole
Department of Paediatric Surgery
Sheffield Children's NHS
Foundation Trust
Sheffield
United Kingdom

Derek Burke
Department of Emergency Medicine
Sheffield Children's NHS
Foundation Trust
Sheffield
United Kingdom

Jill Aylott
Directorate for International MBA
Programmes
International Academy of
Medical Leadership
Sheffield
United Kingdom

ISBN 978-3-319-56223-0 ISBN 978-3-319-56224-7 (eBook)
DOI 10.1007/978-3-319-56224-7

Library of Congress Control Number: 2017944917

Printed on acid-free paper

This Springer imprint is published by Springer Nature
The registered company is Springer International Publishing AG
The registered company address is: Gewerbestrasse 11, 6330 Cham, Switzerland

Foreword

I am delighted to be able to write the foreword for this book because I feel it provides a real insight into the leadership challenges and potential solutions which are facing not just the NHS, but healthcare providers globally.

Rising demand for care, the move towards greater integration and collaboration between health and social care providers and increasing financial constraints are just some of the challenges which today's leaders need to balance alongside the primary focus of ensuring the delivery of safe, high quality care and a positive patient experience.

Today and tomorrow's leaders both clinical and non-clinical will need to add a new suite of skills and approaches to their leadership portfolio if they are to successfully motivate and lead their teams to success given the evolving healthcare landscape. This book explores the theoretical aspects of effective healthcare leadership but more importantly it has practical case studies from experienced clinicians and non-clinicians who are leaders in their own field and who are from a background of clinical medicine, clinical practice and academia.

The book provides an opportunity for fresh thinking, learning and reflection for experienced leaders as well as those just beginning or developing their management careers in the healthcare sector.

Sir Andrew Cash OBE
Chief Executive
Sheffield Teaching Hospitals NHS Foundation Trust
Sheffield, UK

Preface

The primary duty of hospitals globally is to provide patient-centred care that is safe, quality assured, consistent, reliable and cost effective. Whether hospitals are private sector (insurance or self pay based) such as in the USA or public sector (free at point of delivery) for example the NHS in England, hospital executives are constantly challenged to maintain the quality of patient care at an affordable cost.

Hospitals globally face the challenge of managing the delicate interrelationship between finance (money needed to provide the service), performance (delivery of agreed services and targets) and quality (patient safety, outcomes, patient experience), all of which are essential to make hospitals successful.

This book highlights this interrelationship and each chapter takes readers through a journey of the various contributory factors from hospital inquiries that have resulted in hospital failure. Each chapter in turn examines models and approaches to leadership, management, teams and team working, change and overcoming resistance to change and medical leaders as managers. The book relies not only on the theoretical aspects of effective hospital leadership and management but is also supported where appropriate by contemporary case studies. All chapters can be read as stand-alone chapters or in continuity thereby allowing readers to dip in and out of the various topics of interest.

The book will be of interest to hospital executives including experienced, new and budding executives, potential clinical and non-clinical leaders and anyone with an interest in hospital management. The final chapter explores a vision for an increased demand for a future new hybrid role of 'medical leaders' as managers within a world of continuing evolvement of a clinician's 'scope of practice' to enable the evolvement of more patient-centred team working in hospitals and the community. All chapters are written by experienced clinicians and non-clinicians who are leaders in their own field and who are from a background of clinical medicine, clinical practice and academia.

We are very grateful for the support and assistance of Melissa Morton and Andre Tournois from Springer Verlag in the production of this book. We would like to thank the contributors for their timely submission of chapters.

Finally this book would not have been possible without the support of our network of clinician MBA and MSc leaders who have inspired the ideas and content for the chapters and finally to our families and our children whose support has been invaluable.

Sheffield, UK Prasad Godbole
Sheffield, UK Derek Burke
Sheffield, UK Jill Aylott

Contents

1 The Challenge of Context

Derek Burke, Jill Aylott, and Prasad Godbole

1.1 Introduction

The aim of this chapter is to explore the different types of healthcare systems operating globally in terms of the constraints within which they operate and the principles and values which underpin them. The chapter will also review how healthcare systems are predominantly defined by cost, quality and safety. While the principles of these healthcare systems are often espoused and resonate with the public's passion for their healthcare system, the values are often absent in contemporary debate. Regardless of the healthcare context there is a consensus that the healthcare systems have to change in order to improve [1–3] as variation in outcomes continues to be seen within and between countries [4]. Improvements in healthcare are more likely to succeed when led by clinicians rather than managers [3] and must be undertaken in partnership with patients, families [5, 6] and local communities [7]. In 2011, Sweden enacted a new patient safety law which offers everyone affected by healthcare—patients, consumers and health workers the opportunity to influence the health care system. This Swedish initiative should inspire those operating health care systems globally to strive to improve patient safety.

D. Burke
Department of Emergency Medicine, Sheffield Children's NHS Foundation Trust, Sheffield, UK
e-mail: derek.burke@sch.nhs.uk

J. Aylott
Directorate for International MBA Programmes, International Academy of Medical Leadership, Sheffield, UK
e-mail: Jill.Aylott@iamedicalleadership.com

P. Godbole (✉)
Department of Paediatric Surgery, Sheffield Children's NHS Foundation Trust, Sheffield, UK
e-mail: Prasad.Godbole@sch.nhs.uk

1.2 Global Healthcare Systems

Healthcare systems may be funded privately, publicly or by a combination of both. They may be 'not for profit' or for profit. The healthcare system may be insurance based, with patients relying on their private health insurance or be free at the point of delivery (e.g. the National Health Service (NHS) in the United Kingdom which is funded centrally from taxation) or a combination of the two. In the USA, the introduction of the Affordable Care Act as federal law has seen a shift towards the concept of universal healthcare.

Irrespective of the system of healthcare in place, the values and principles that guide the system remain similar (see Table 1.1). A study undertaken in Iran [9] developed a conceptual framework for quality of care from interviews with 700 stakeholders, who came up with similar domains to Maxwell [10]; IOM [8] and the WHO [7] but included 'empathy' as a core value in defining the quality of health care.

P. Godbole et al. (eds.), *Why Hospitals Fail*, DOI 10.1007/978-3-319-56224-7_1

Table 1.1 Values and principles guiding healthcare systems

US [8]	WHO [7]	Mosadeghrad [9]	Maxwell [10]
Safe	Safe	Efficacy	Acceptability
Efficient	Efficient	Efficiency	Efficiency
Effective	Effective	Effectiveness	
Patient centered	Patient centred	Empathy	Relevance
Timely Equitable	Accessible Equitable	Environment	Accessible Equitable

In systems underpinned by private healthcare such as in the USA, the ability to pay plays an important part in the decision of individuals to access healthcare.

In government funded systems such as the NHS further principles form the core values on which the system has been developed

- that it meet the needs of everyone
- that it be free at the point of delivery
- that it be based on clinical need, not ability to pay

- Working together for patients
- Respect and dignity
- Compassion

Hospitals across the globe have a common set of strategic objectives which can be mapped to the following three domains:

- Finance
- Delivery
- Experience

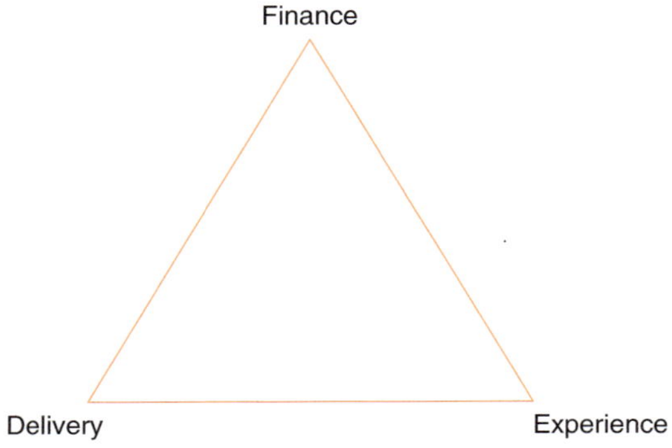

Diagram of the Finance/Delivery/Experience triad

Table 1.2 Domains important for patient safety practice interventions [11]

• Safety culture, teamwork and leadership development
• Structural organisational characteristics (e.g. size, organisational complexity)
• External factors (e.g. financial or performance incentives or patient safety regulations)
• Availability of implementation and management tools (e.g. training resources or internal organisational incentives)

An understanding of how these objectives are managed and how they interact with one another will form the basis for an understanding of the organisational factors which cause some hospitals to fail. When we use the term fail in the context of this book we are talking of failure in relation to patient safety, rather than service delivery or finance. Taylor et al. [11] argue that the role of context and how it affects patient safety interventions needs to be better understood. The authors describe a taxonomy of four broad domains of contextual features important for patient safety practice interventions (see Table 1.2).

In relation to a 'safety culture' employees are guided by an organisation-wide commitment to safety in which each member upholds their own safety norms and those of their coworkers [11, 12]. Practical ways of engaging the team in the development of a 'safety culture' are to work through patient safety checklists for example the Manchester Patient safety Checklist [18].

We will consider how an undue focus on delivering financial and service delivery domain objectives can lead to devastating failures in patient safety.

Whatever the current mood music says about the central role of quality in healthcare, finance remains the pre-eminent domain. Where hospitals and healthcare systems are centrally funded, the resources available to deliver healthcare are dictated by central government: whereas in a free market economy demand primarily determines the resources available.

These three domains will be considered in turn and details of financial and economic theories to support this will be discussed in more detail in following sections.

1.3 Finance

It is important for any hospital to be able to maintain financial security to enable delivery of high quality, safe, patient care. It remains a challenge to many Directors of Finance to balance the books and at the same time invest in areas that improve patient care. Finance in a hospital in its simplest form deals with a quantitative parameter: money, which can be represented by the graph below.

All hospitals are required to break even at the end of the financial year to balance the books. In addition they may seek to generate a surplus to fund new developments and where hospitals are 'for profit', to provide returns for their investors and shareholders. The balance between income and expenditure determines how much cash a hospital has available…cash is what makes the hospital run.

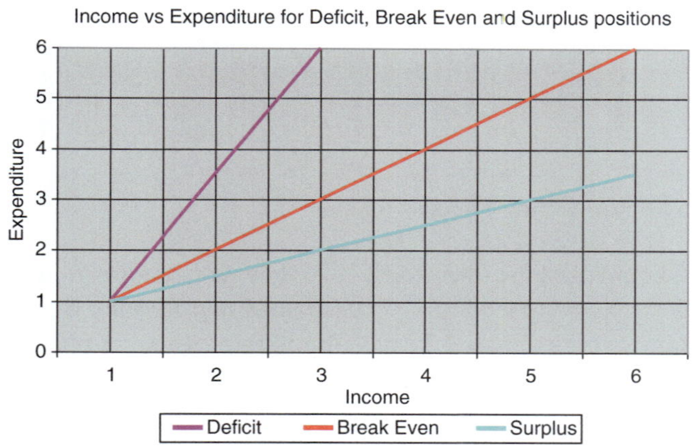

Graph of income vs expenditure and deficit, surplus and break even

We can summarise the finance domain as being the bottom right hand corner of a real time spread sheet of the hospital's financial position: black is good, red is bad.

1.4 Delivery

There are two components to delivery:

- Activity
- Targets

1.5 Activity

Activity refers to all of the work undertaken which generates income. This is predominantly clinical activity such as patient episodes in the emergency department (ED), out-patient department (OPD) and theatres. There are other non-clinical activities which generate income such as training and research, which we will not consider further here.

Capacity and demand also feature here. Capacity defines the maximum activity we can undertake when demand is not a constraining factor. It has three components: absolute capacity; the maximum activity we can manage within the current resources working at maximum efficiency and effectiveness, ignoring constraints due to the need to continue delivering targets; the maximum activity we can manage with the current systems in place, ignoring constraints due to the need to continue delivering targets and the maximum activity we can manage with the current systems in place while continuing to deliver targets. Current demand defines the maximum activity we can deliver when there are no capacity constraints. Experience has shown that when we remove the demand regulators (e.g. waiting times in ED and waiting lists in in-patients) demand increases. There is also the phenomenon of provider induced demand "If we build it they will come," e.g. In the NHS in the U.K. The NHS Direct service was set up as a service catering for patients to ring for advice for non emergency conditions. This had a minimal impact on demand for current emergency care services but created a new demand.

Activity has two components:

- Action: that component of activity which generates income
- Waste: that component of activity which does not attract income; waste can also occur when processes are duplicated. This is often referred to in improvement science as a key determinant to improving services and will be discussed later in this chapter.

Note that a considerable amount of waste contributes to the quality of a service as perceived by the patient, even if it does not attract income e.g. patients referred to an admitting team by the emergency department who, following a wait for several hours for review are subsequently discharged attract a charge for that referral.

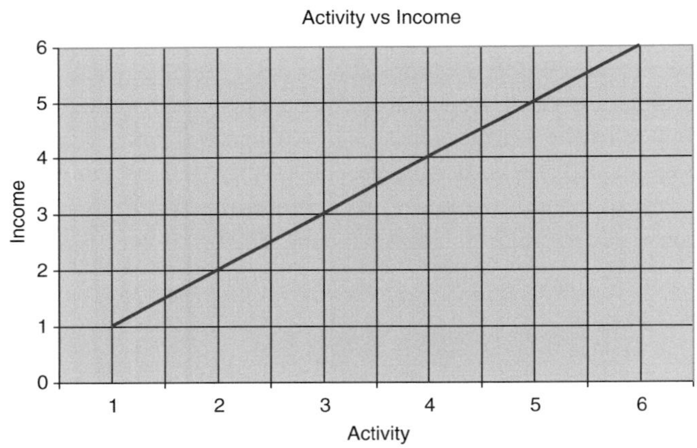

Graph of activity vs income

Activity can be summarised by the graph above.

An increase in activity results in an increase in income. So activity, like finance, deals with qualitative parameters, money and patient episodes. Not all activity is clinically relevant; Porter and Lee [13] argue activity must be valued by the end user/patient in terms of future costing models. This can lead to an element of 'gaming' when priority is given to activity on the basis of income generation income rather than prioritising patient defined quality activity.

How we choose to deliver activity is constrained by targets. Again depending on the healthcare system in place, these targets may be set by individual hospital boards for their executive team or by governments. Targets are externally mandated performance indicators, the delivery of which are generally linked to income (i.e. failure to meet a target can result in a financial penalty to the organisation or to individual members of the executive team). Targets such as the 18 week referral to treatment target in the NHS can influence how we manage activity and may, in some circumstances, distort those priorities.

There are five ways we can influence activity:

- Keep activity the same but deliver it at additional cost:
  - Expenditure, either by increasing the resource required to deliver activity and targets or make improvements in the quality of the service which do not impact on delivery
- Increase activity at no additional cost:
  - Efficiency: doing more with the same resources or the same with less resource.
  - Effectiveness: not doing that which does not work (e.g. ineffective drugs or treatments)
- Increase activity at additional cost:
  - Expanding the volume of current activity: spending money to do more of what we currently do
  - Extending the scope of activity: taking on new activity (e.g. new services)

In reality we use a combination of the five.

No matter how efficient or effective an organisation is, there will always be waste (e.g. sickness) As resources become scarce and less money is available to fund healthcare, there will be a high vacancy rates, work related stress, staff sickness and dissatisfaction which will impact upon patient safety and quality [14]. The presence of waste provides opportunites for leading and developing service improvement projects. Research shows that many start an improvement project but fewer finish successfully with even fewer developing a shared and sustained capacity in their service to make and lead improvement [2]. It is often the absence of leadership that leads to failures in service improvement projects.

The following table summarises the relationship between the finance and delivery domains:

The finance/deliver matrix

		Finance	
		–	+
Delivery	–	–	–
	+	–	+

When the delivery domain fails to perform to plan it will always attribute that failure to a lack of the resources required to deliver or to those resources being released too late in the financial year to impact on performance. The four permutations are:

- Delivery fails: finance succeeds: finance has failed to release resources required to delivery to perform, finance are to blame for sitting on the resources required by delivery to do their job.
- Delivery succeeds: finance fails: finance has failed to adequately manage the finances.
- Delivery fails: finance fails: finance has failed to adequately manage the finances and as a consequence did not provide sufficient resource for delivery to perform.
- Delivery succeeds: finance succeeds: that's the job.

In all adverse scenarios the blame for failure is attributed to the finance department. Finance is always hostage to delivery. Conversely delivery will always preferentially draw down money from finance (expand or extend) rather than transform (efficiency or effectiveness); drawing down money is easy and transformation difficult.

1.6 Experience

Experience is sub-divided into quality and patient safety. These will be considered in turn.

1.7 Quality

Quality is such a value laden term (good quality, poor quality) that it would be better to substitute it with another neutral term such as standard. But the term is so deeply embedded in modern healthcare parlance that we will have to accept its use, but always with the rider that when it is used we require a specific definition of the meaning of the term in that specific context. Quality is now understood as being a multi-dimensional concept in relation to healthcare quality. Donabedian [15] explores quality in relation to Structure, (refers to attributes of the healthcare setting to deliver the care) Process (covers all elements of delivering health care and relates to the interpersonal connection between patients and families and health workers) and Outcomes is the end result of the healthcare intervention.

For the purpose of this chapter quality is defined as performing to a defined standard in relation to Structure, Process and Outcome.

We will examine the relationship between quality and standards by starting with performance. Performance is what we do; it denotes the globality of our activity. We cannot measure all of what we do, so we pick some components of what we do to measure. These we call performance indicators. Not all performance is considered as valued by the end user but it might be identified as clinically relevant. To address this issue, Øvretveit [16] identified healthcare quality on three dimensions: professional, client and management quality. Darzi [5] supported this with his definition of quality in relation to being clinically effective, personal and safe.

If we agree a specific level of performance to be delivered (using a specific performance indicator as the metric) this is called a standard. If we perform to that standard that activity we can be said to have met our quality standard. So quality becomes an objective parameter defined according to a standard which is defined by measuring a specific performance indicator. Not all performance is considered as valued by the end user but it might be identified as clinically relevant. To address this issue, Øvretveit [16] identified healthcare quality on three dimensions: professional, client and management quality. Darzi [5] supported this with his definition of quality in relation to being clinically effective, personal and safe. If standards are central to quality how do we derive the standard to meet?

When we set a standard, that standard may be derived empirically, by consensus or it may be evidence based; few current standards are evidenced based. Note that there are many aspects of medicine where there are no standards in place so it is difficult to measure quality. This means that there is a need for doctors to develop skills in inductive processes to use leadership skills to generate knowledge from a consensus in practice. Having set our standard, whether it is empirically or consensus derived or evidence based, we then need to monitor compliance against that standard to ensure that we are delivering a quality service.

The process of monitoring compliance is called audit. There are three means by which we can ensure compliance:

Quality control: measuring compliance against the standard after the event.
Quality assurance: measuring compliance against the standard during the event
Total quality management: compliance becomes a real time process of interdicting issues which would lead to non-compliance with the standard, i.e. the improvement is embedded within the system delivering the performance, i.e., getting it right first time.

The audit cycle is the process by which we measure compliance against the standard. The following diagram illustrates the interrelationship between the audit cycle and research.

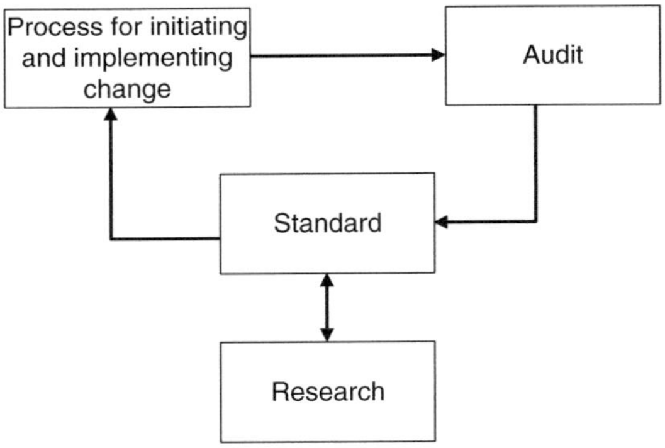

Targets are also standards but are standards which are externally mandated; quality is an internally set standard. Quality is what we set as a standard to meet; targets are what "they" set as a standard to meet.

We need to be clear that not everything we should measure is measurable, similarly there is a risk that when we choose performance indicators we will make important what we measure, rather than measure what is important. Or to paraphrase John Lingle [20] 'What gets measured gets done.' So the setting of national targets has the potential to distort local priorities and potentially compromise patient safety as local needs give way to nationally mandated needs.

As noted above Activity and Finance are easy to measure, some of the elements of experience (quality and safety) are not.

The dilemma is to know how to capture that which is important that we cannot measure: "can we measure it and if not how do we capture it?" There are new developments to explore how 'soft intelligence' can be used for healthcare quality and safety [17]. The authors suggest complimentary ways such as *Aggregation*, pulling together a sample of patient stories to see if there are any common themes; *Triangulation*, to identify how strands of data support each other and *Instrumentalization* how data from carers and patients might be more useful to support an argument premised on quantitative data to help persuade others for the need for improvement.

1.8 Patient Safety

Patients are safe when they are not coming to harm as a result of our acts of commission (things we do) or omission (things we fail to do); patient safety is a culture which strives to eliminate preventable healthcare associated harm (Table 1.3).

Harm can be defined as any physical, psychological or mental impairment resulting from a healthcare associated adverse event. Harm can lead to:

- Death
- Permanent impairment
- Temporary impairment
- No harm my occur

Table 1.3 Example of unpreventable and preventable healthcare associated harm

Unpreventable healthcare associated harm A previously healthy patient with no previous history of exposure to penicillin is given IV benzylpenicillin for severe community acquired pneumonia and suffers an anaphylactic reaction.
Preventable healthcare associated harm The same patient re-attends a few weeks later and is admitted, gives a history of a previous anaphylactic reaction to penicillin but due to poor note keeping and checking before administration of IV penicillin suffers an anaphylactic reaction.

Adverse events are any unplanned events which may result in harm to patients. Note that most adverse events do not result in harm.

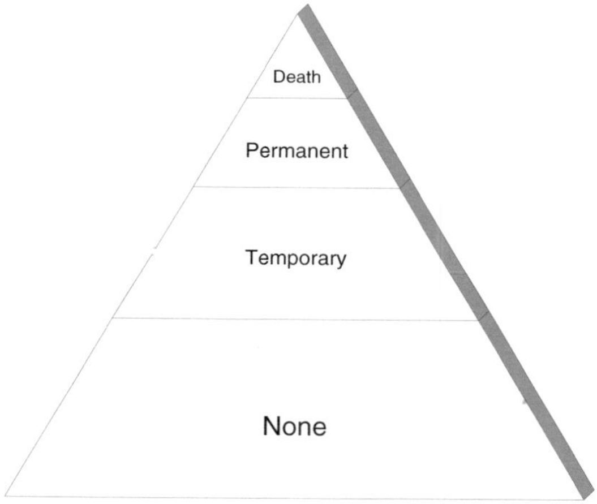

Hierarch and frequency of adverse events

Deaths due to adverse events are rare; the most common outcome from an adverse event is no harm which comprises over 90% of all incidents reported. We call adverse events which do not result in harm triggers. Triggers are important because they give us intelligence on factors which may result in future harm.

Adverse events are caused by:

- Errors of judgement: cognitive failures
- Process failures: psychomotor failures
- Violations: affective failures
- Hazards

The terms used are pejorative but are not intended to be as most adverse events are unintended.

We can summarise the relationship between patient safety, adverse events, harm and triggers:

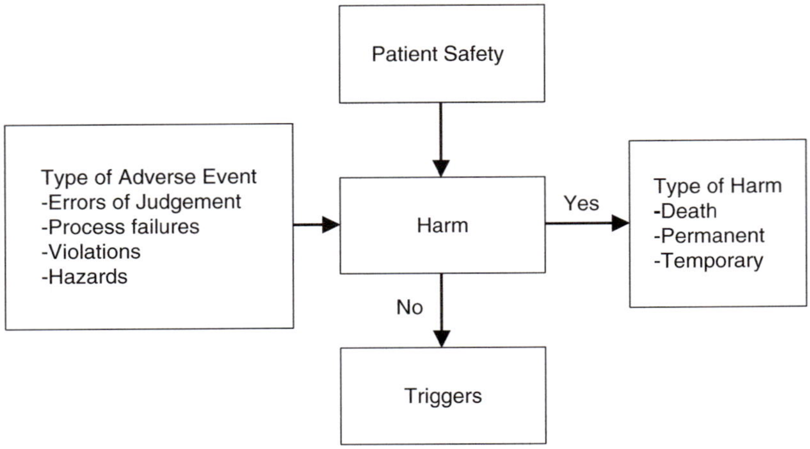

1.8.1 How Do We Prevent Harm to Patients?

We prevent harm to patients by understanding which adverse events are causing or posing a risk to patient safety and putting in place measures to prevent them from occurring or by mitigating the effect of those adverse events. The key to this is reporting and analysing adverse events when they occur. We can also promote a more proactive emergence of a patient safety culture, by developing much more awareness of patient safety in teams throughout the organisation.

Before we go on to consider the reporting system we will consider risk. Risk is the likelihood (probability) of an adverse event causing harm multiplied by the consequence. To allow us to quantify risk a matrix has been developed which gives a numerical value to the severity of various types of consequence (e.g. harm to patients, financial loss, etc.). The following matrix is based on the National Patient Safety Agency (NPSA 2006) UK model (Table 1.4).

The degree of risk (on a scale of 1–25) dictates the speed of response. We may decide that a risk is such that it should be prevented, or that we can mitigate the effect of the risk to bring it down to a level that is acceptable (less than 5 is conventional).

The diagram below summarises the process which we will discuss:

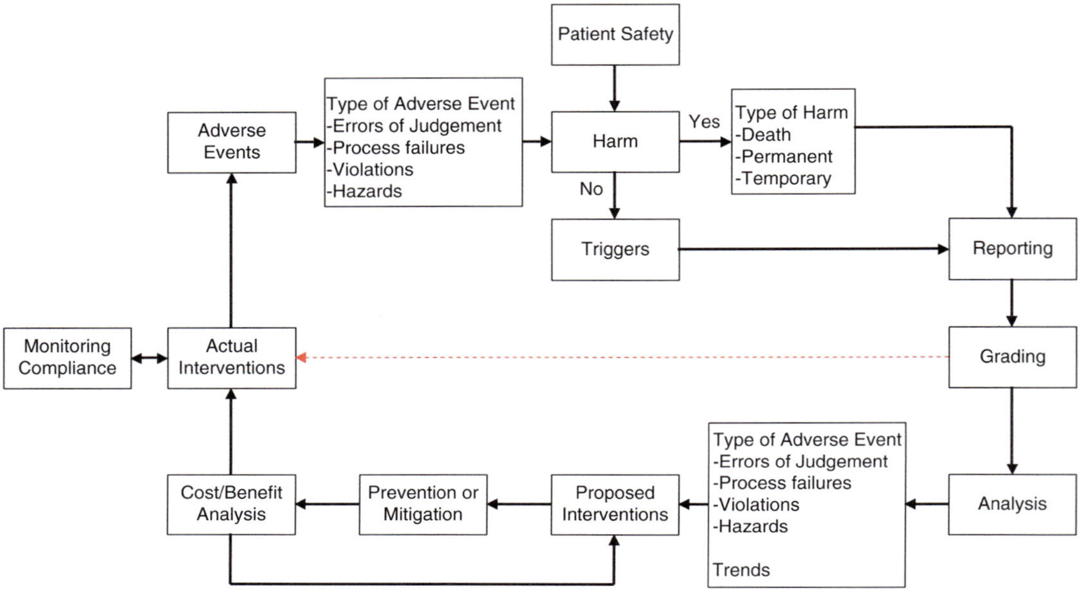

Table 1.4 Risk matrix (National Patient Safety Agency—U.K.)

Consequence (C) =		Likelihood (L) =		Rating (C × L) =	
Consequence			Likelihood		
1	Negligible	Very minor injury/none or minor treatment/adverse health outcome/some disruption to service/minor financial loss/potential for public concern	1	Rare	May occur/recur only in exceptional circumstances (not expected to occur for years)
2	Minor	Minor injury/<3 days off work/adverse health outcome/short term disruption to service/minor financial loss or claim <£10,000/local media coverage	2	Unlikely	Could occur/recur at some time (expected to occur annually)
3	Moderate	Medium injury/4–14 days off work/adverse health outcome/moderate service disruption/moderate financial loss or claim £10,000 – £100,000/local media coverage long term	3	Possible	Loss might occur/recur at some time (expected to occur monthly)
4	Major	Permanent injury or disability/closure of a service/major financial loss or claim £100,000 – £1M/possible litigation/National media coverage short term	4	Likely	Will probably occur/recur in most circumstances (expected to occur weekly)
5	Catastrophic	Death(s)/multiple permanent injury or health effects/extended service disruption or closure/Financial loss or claim >£1M/National media coverage long term	5	Almost certain	Is expected to occur/recur in most circumstances (expected to occur daily)
15–25 = Extreme	Extreme risk, immediate action required		8–12 = High	High risk, action planned immediately, commenced within 1 month	
4–6 = Moderate	Moderate risk, action planned within 1 month, commenced within 3 months		1–3 = Low	Low risk, action planned within 3 months, reviewed within 1 year	

"Source: Modified form the NPSA risk matrix" and reference (for the complete version:see the below link): http://www.npsa.nhs.uk/nrls/improvingpatientsafety/patient-safety-tools-and-guidance/risk-assessment-guides/risk-matrix-for-risk-managers/

Adverse events are reported using the Incident Reporting form or web based incident reporting platforms. These forms are collated and reviewed on a regular (usually weekly) basis and graded using the risk matrix. Very high risks (>15) will normally be addressed immediately (see red dotted line). Risks are analysed to determine the cause; this analysis may be informal, taking place at the risk grading meeting, or may be more formal through a root cause analysis. It is helpful when analysing the risk to classify the type of adverse event as the type of adverse event will suggest the actions required. Once the cause of the risk is ascertained an intervention is proposed. This intervention may be designed to prevent or to mitigate the risk.

Prevention

Latex allergy is a specific risk in hospitals. Many hospitals have now moved towards becoming latex free to remove the risk of latex allergy due to procedural gloves.

Mitigation

IV potassium errors have resulted in a number of deaths, but it is difficult to completely remove IV potassium from clinical areas. Most hospital mitigate the risk by restricting IV potassium vials to a few high usage areas and treating IV potassium as a Controlled drug.

The intervention is subject to a cost/benefit analysis, if the cost of the proposed intervention is considered too high compared to the benefit, the proposed intervention is reviewed. There are many risks on a hospital risk register and insufficient funds to prevent all of them so in most cases risks are mitigated (i.e. brought down to an acceptable level of risk through a reasonable expendit ure of money or resources).

Implementation of the intervention must be monitored to ensure compliance. The loop is closed by monitoring the outcome to determine if the incidence of the adverse outcome is increasing, remaining the same or falling.

The relationship between risk and patient safety is summarised below:

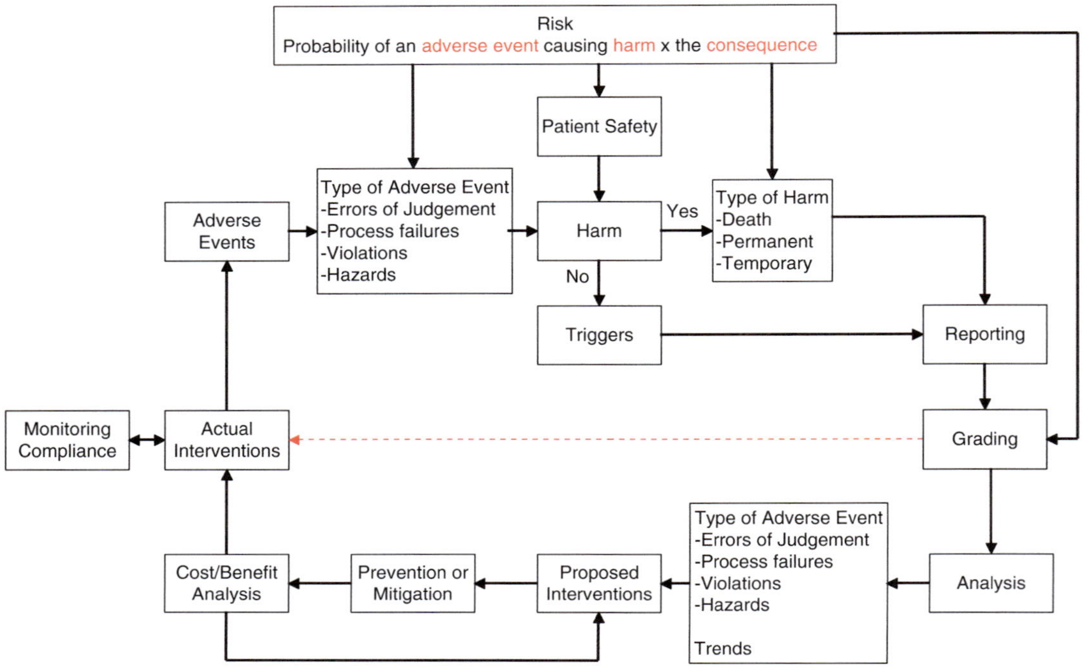

So we now have an understanding of the components of the three domains which we can summarise in Figure below.

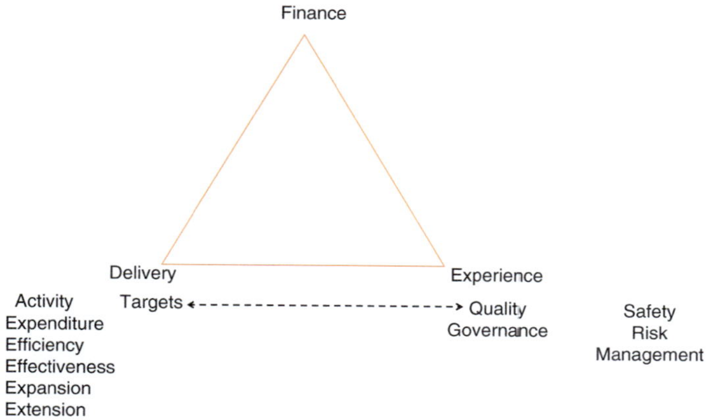

How do we balance the competing needs of finance and delivery, both measured quantitatively, with experience?

1.9 Board Assurance Framework

Most if not all hospitals and organisations will have a hospital Board which comprise executive and non-executive directors. The non-executive directors are tasked with taking an overview of the organisation and for gaining assurance that the hospital is meeting its duties, principally delivering on the three domains. The diagram below summarises how the board assurance framework is related to the three domains and their sub-domains:

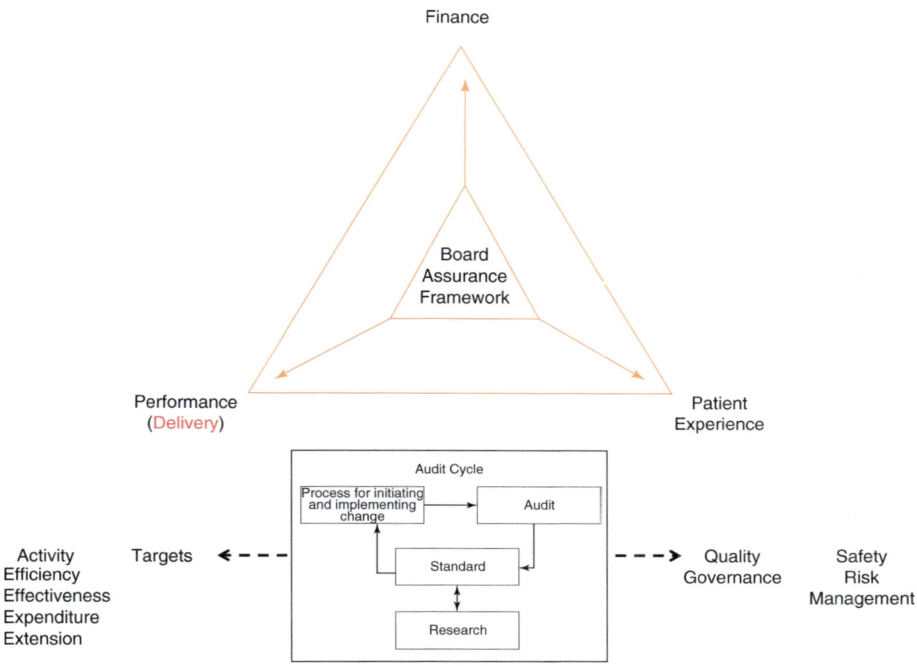

The purpose of the framework is to balance the conflicting demands of finance, delivery and experience to ensure the trust meets it financial duties, delivers on its targets while keeping patients safe.

Despite this framework there are still major failures in hospitals where patient safety is compromised [19]. This is evidenced by the litigations and the data held relating to this litigation suggests human error occurs and will still occur. It is also expensive to hospitals when things go wrong and often clinical staff are blamed by being singled out as the cause of the error when health care is delivered within a system/team. The problem is determining when patient safety is deteriorating. In general the metrics which indicate a significant level of deterioration in patient safety in a hospital relate to the higher levels of harm such as multiple patient deaths or patients suffering permanent harm. Hospitals seem to find it difficult to detect significant changes in the lower levels of harm which pre-date the higher levels of harm. Why is this?

If we return to the three domains for a moment to consider how we detect problems with each domain this will shed light on the major problem with pre-empting major failures of patient safety.

Recall that finance is the bottom right hand corner of the spreadsheet, red is bad, black is good. If there is good financial control and timely data on income and expenditure, then finances should rarely become an issue without the hospital being aware of the problem evolving over a period of time; giving them the opportunity to rectify the problem (see below however on timely data).

The position is similar for delivery. Activity is the bottom right hand corner of a spreadsheet and is measured according to actual activity against planned activity and income. Red is bad, black is good. Activity and income are related. As with finance if there is good quality timely data on activity and income then activity, which derives most of a hospital's income, should rarely become an issue without the management team being aware of the problem evolving over a period of time; giving them the opportunity to rectify the problem (as for finance see below on timely data).

The comments above relate also to quality, where we use the definition of quality proposed in this paper of quality being performance to standard. Standards are those components of the globality of the hospital activity which can be measured or otherwise quantified. Not all elements that are considered to contribute to the more generic concept of quality (in terms of values such as "this is a good service," "this is a bad service") can be measured. The problem arises if these more qualitative parameters are important contributors to patient safety. Two examples:

- We know that nursing levels on wards are an important predictor of patient safety, although there is no evidence base for the precise numbers. Nonetheless we can use expert consensus to establish levels which are considered safe and set these levels as standard to assess quality against.
- The culture within a group of staff will mitigate for shortages of staff where there are strong values and a good team culture. We can measure the effectiveness of team dynamics and organisational cultures, but to do so is challenging. Staff shortages can be mitigated by positive value sets and team dynamic, whereas in a team with poor dynamic and weak values, even when staffing levels meeting consensus standard levels may compromise patient safety.

This goes back to the mantra of ensuring we measure what is important rather than making important what we can measure.

1.10 Relationship Between Cost, Quality and Safety

While the relation between income and expenditure and activity and income is linear, the relationship between quality and cost, safety and cost and quality and safety is non-linear. The graph below summarise the relationship between quality and cost and safety and cost.

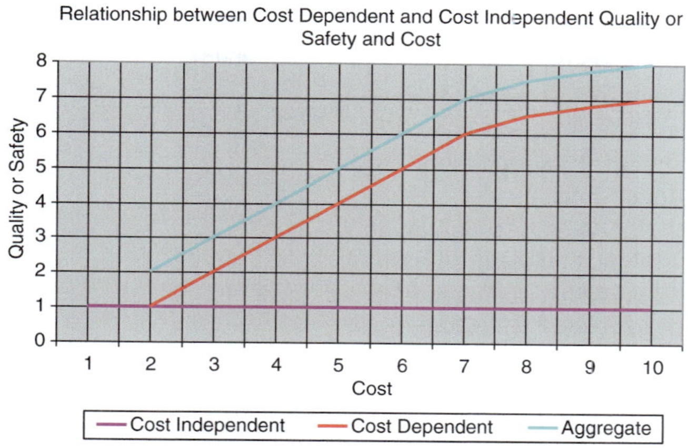

Note that even with no cost there is a basic level of quality or safety. We call this cost-independent quality or safety (e.g. employing nice people costs the same as employing nasty people but customers or patients feel that the quality of the service is better and nice people will likely have stronger values and be better team members). For some aspects of quality there is a linear relationship between quality or safety and cost, e.g. employing more nurses or cleaners, each adds to the quality or safety in a linear fashion, we call this cost-dependent quality or safety. Note however that there comes a point of diminishing returns where increasing costs leads to a diminishing return on quality and safety return (the cost of wine is generally related to the quality of the wine, but for the average wine drinker a $500 bottle of wine will not be perceived as giving the same quantum of quality improvement over a $50 bottle of wine than the quantum of quality improvement of a $50 bottle of wine would give over a $5 bottle of wine).In reality the relationship between quality or safety and cost follows the aggregate line, where there is a basic cost independent level of quality or safety followed by a near linear relationship between cost and level of quality or safety and cost, followed by a region where the improvement in quality or cost diminishes with increasing cost.

So if we summarise the relationship between quality or safety and cost:

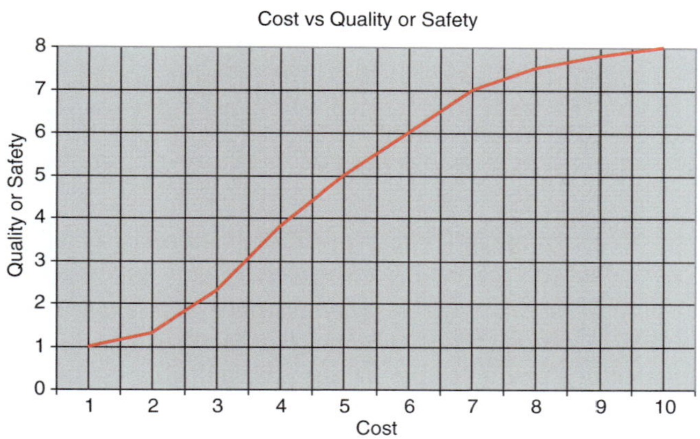

The relationship between cost and quality and cost and safety is non-linear. There is in addition, a relationship between quality and safety. This relationship is complex as both quality and safety have cost dependent and cost independent elements, so to express the relationship between quality and safety we need to take account of the inter-relationship between cost, quality and safety. This involves looking at the relationship in three dimensions.

When determining the axes to assign each parameter to, we must be clear that both cost and quality are independent variables (although with an inter-dependency) in that we can decide the level of quality we wish to deliver (within overall income constraints) and also decide how much cost we wish to expend on various interventions (again within overall income constraints). This would place cost and quality on the x and z axis and safety on the y axis, as safety is dependent on the amount we expend on quality. Which of the two, quality or cost, is the principle driver depends on the economic state, where money is plentiful quality drives the agenda, where money is in short supply cost drives the agenda. One of the questions to consider is whether it is the professionals that determine the level of quality without consultation with patients? Experience based design is more likely to get the quality embedded first time 'right first time' when patients are at the helm, telling us how they define quality and what is important to them.

So we can express the relationship between cost, quality and safety in three dimensions, with cost and quality on the x and z axis respectively (the independent variables, although they have a co-dependency) and safety on the y axis (the dependent variable):

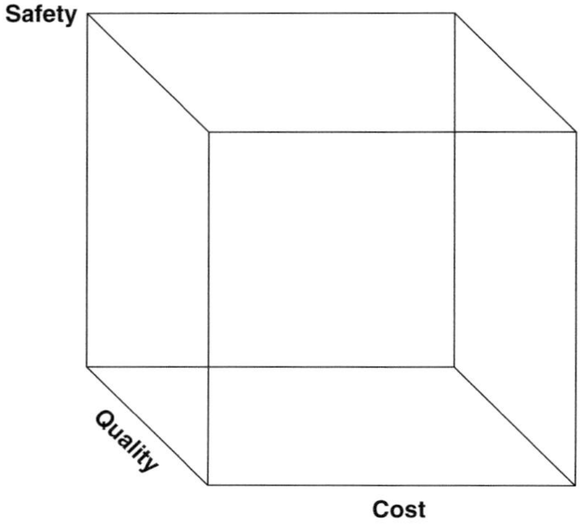

We now add in the relationship between quality and cost:

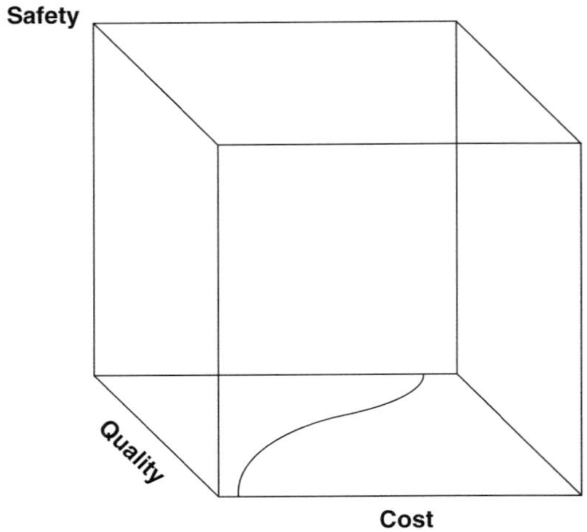

Then add in the relationship between quality and safety:

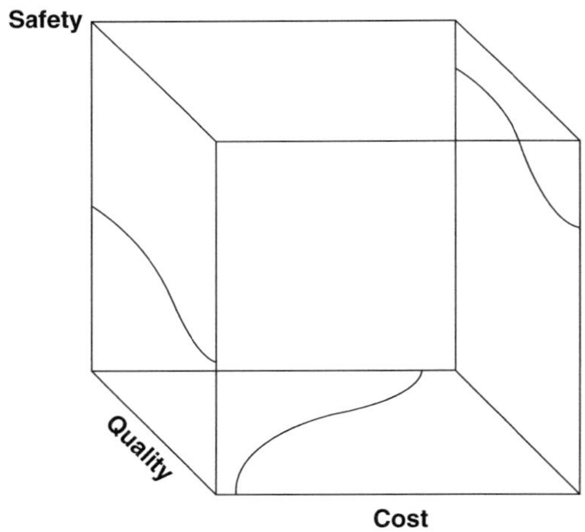

There are two lines for the relationship between quality and safety: one to the left of the graph when cost is low, where the overall safety level is low and one to the right of the graph where cost is high, where the overall safety level is high. We finally add in the relationship between cost and safety:

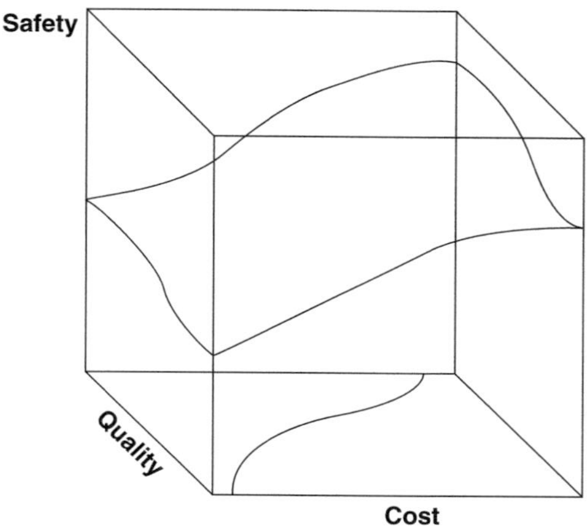

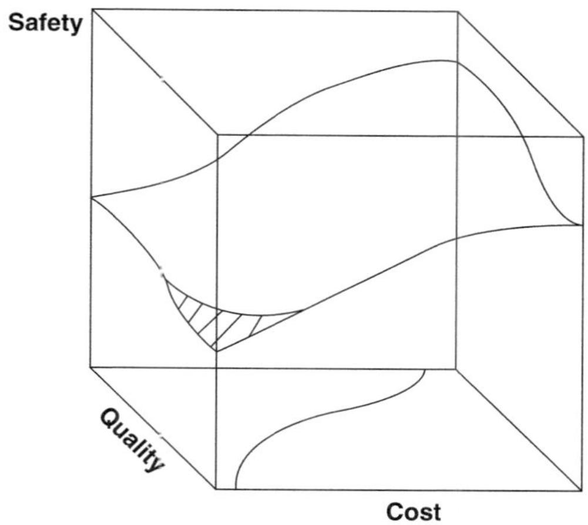

Again we can see that there are two lines, one to the back of the graph, where for any level of cost safety is higher and one to the front of the graph, where for any level of cost safety is lower. The level of safety for any specific cost is variable and dependent on the choices we make about the quality initiatives we fund; make the wrong choices and expenditure is wasted on initiatives which give a low return of safety for a given cost (e.g. buying more nursing time is likely to result in a greater impact on patient safety than building a new hospital entrance atrium). Once these lines are drawn we can see that we have a landscape the contours of which describe the level of safety for any combination of cost and quality.

When we consider the relationship between quality, safety and cost we can see that there are a number of areas of the safety landscape which are unlikely to occur:

Low cost, low quality and low safety will exist together but due to the non-cost dependent component of quality and safety will not reach zero, in a similar fashion we would never have a zero cost health system. So we will modify the graph to reflect this:

High cost and low quality are unlikely to co-exist as in a regulated healthcare system the checks in the system would mean that we would rarely be permitted to select such a poor choice of quality initiatives to fund (but note that in major capital schemes costs can overrun considerably and effectively lead to such a situation). So we will modify the graph to reflect this:

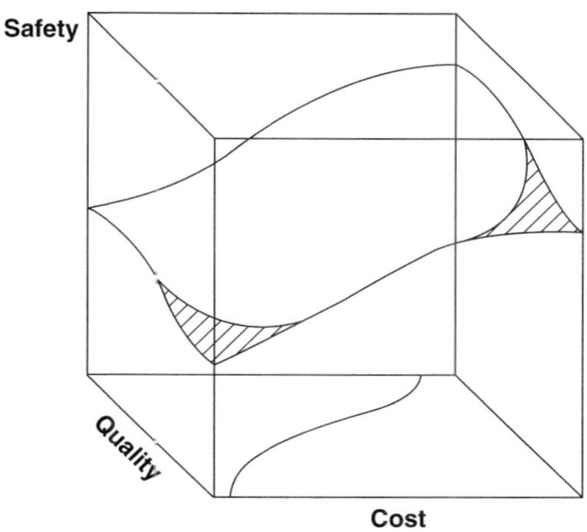

Low cost and high quality are less likely to exist as cost dependent quality (the predominant type of quality) costs money so the graph is modified to reflect this:

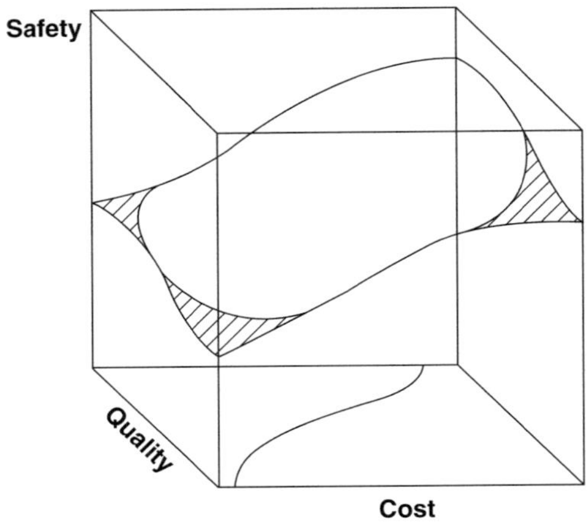

So we now have a landscape which qualitatively describes the inter-relationship between quality, safety and cost and demonstrates that for any level of cost and quality there is an expected level of safety to be achieved. At high cost and high quality, safety is high, at low cost and low quality, safety is low.

We can abstract this safety landscape from the graph:

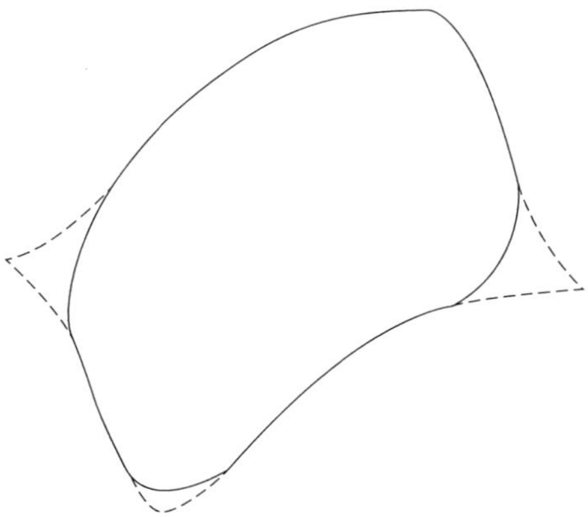

And use it to qualitatively represent the safety landscape in a number of ways:

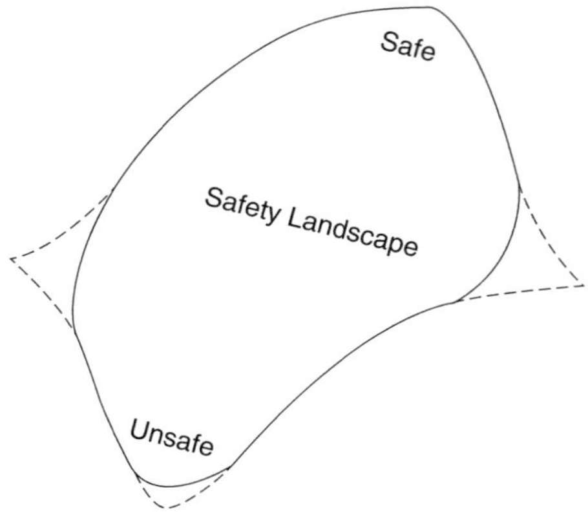

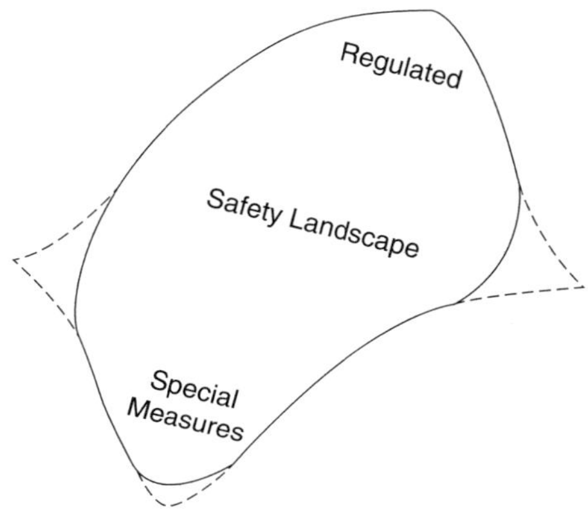

1.11 Event—Action—Outcome Lag:

Managing systems effectively is predicated on having timely information to determine actions and then implementing those actions in a timely manner such that the actions relate to the condition that drove the actions. There are two problems:

1. Information systems in hospitals are often (but not always) poorly developed to derive real time information on the current state.
2. Even when current information is available there is often a lag between that receipt of that information and the decision as to what action to take and implementing those actions, with the result that the conditions may have changed and the actions chosen may not be appropriate to those conditions, meaning at best the actions are ineffective or at worse they actually make the situation worse.

3. Even if current information is available the situation may be novel meaning that ad hoc actions will be developed empirically.

A good analogy is a car going into a skid. The information coming to the driver is often delayed leading to over-reaction and exacerbation of the skid. Experienced drivers "learn" that the counter-intuitive actions of pumping the brakes and turning into the skid are the correct actions. These counter-intuitive actions could not be rationally derived in real time in the heat of the moment, but have to be learnt.

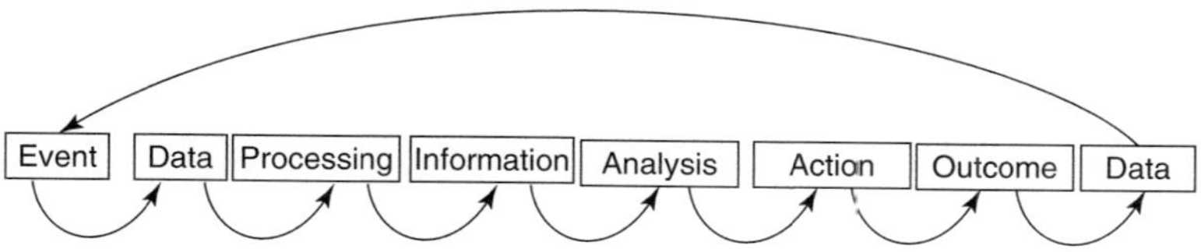

If we examine this on the safety landscape it becomes clearer. An organisation starts at point on the safety landscape A then moves to B as an unintended consequence of a cost cutting exercise. The move is detected and the cycle above begins. The dotted line from B to A shows the intended outcome of the corrective action, but because there is a time lag in recognising the unintended consequence, determining the corrective action and implementing that action, the situation has changed adversely to C. By the time this is detected and the cycle implemented to put in place the corrective action to bring the situation back to normal (demonstrated by the dotted line from C to A) the situation has deteriorated further to D. So the time lag means that in a dynamic state, the interventions to correct the situation may have no effect because they are acting on a new situation or at worse could make that situation worse:

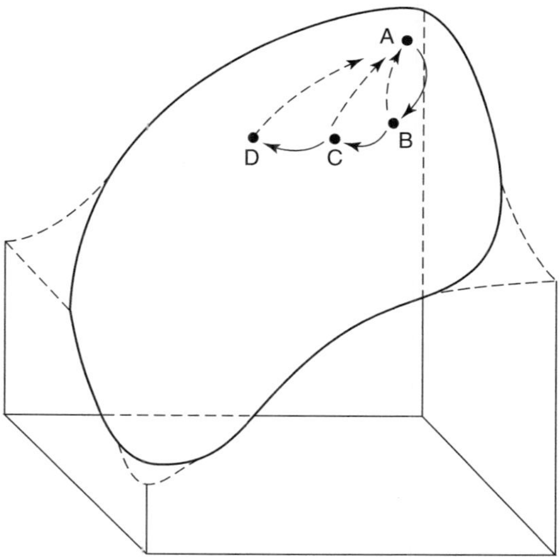

We can now consider how patient safety can deteriorate catastrophically with little notice.

The diagram below show that when finances are tight (e.g. the current economic recession) or a hospital moves into a more rigidly managed system (e.g. in centrally regulated healthcare systems) the requirement to meet financial duties has the potential to impact on patient care. Delivery will continue to preferentially draw down money rather than transform and since both delivery and finance are measured quantitatively delivery can demonstrate that it is failing. Delivery will attribute this failure to finance failing to release sufficient money to provide the resources that delivery requires so money is drawn down from finance (red arrow). The only option for finance is to draw money down from other areas (pale arrow). There is an invisible flow of money from those areas where we cannot measure the impact i.e. experience, because we cannot directly see the effect in a quantitative way, the degree of underfunding of these areas will only show when there are major failures in patient safety.

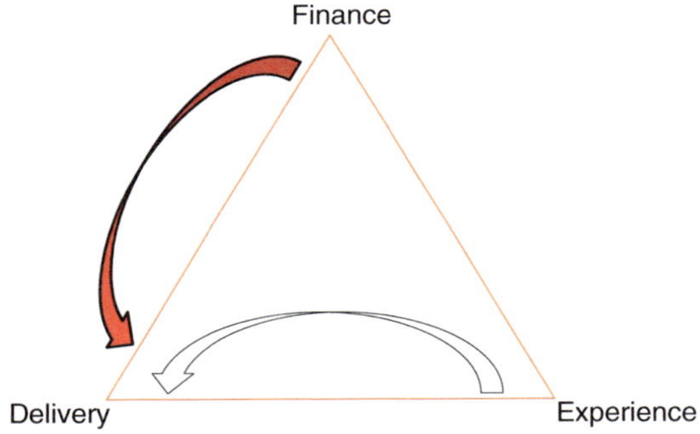

Diagram of Finance/Delivery/Experience Triad demonstrating how catastrophic deterioration can occur

1.12 Summary

The above discussion sets the scene and the context within which hospitals work. Success or failure of a hospital is judged by the aforementioned parameters. However there are many other contributory factors and variables that can make or break a hospital. Subsequent chapters will address these variables in more detail.

References

1. Berwick D, Nolan TW, Whittington J. The triple aim: care, health and cost: the remaining barriers to integrated care are not technical; they are political. Health Aff. 2008;27(3):759–69.
2. Øvretveit J. Improvement leaders: what do they and should they do? A summary of a review of research. Qual Saf Healhcare. 2010;19:490–2.
3. Øvretveit J, Andreen-Sachs M, Carlsson J, Gustafsson H, Hansson J, Keller C, Lofgren S, Mazzocato P, Tolf S, Brommels M. Implementing organisation and management innovations in Swedish healthcare: lessons from a comparison of 12 cases. J Health Organ Manag. 2012;26(2):237–57.
4. Kossarova L, Blunt I, Bradsley M. Quality watch, focus on: international comparisons of healthcare quality, what can the UK learn? London: The Health Foundation and Nuffield Trust; 2015.
5. Darzi A. High quality care for all. London: Department of Health; 2008.
6. Institute for Healthcare Improvement. Achieving the vision of excellence in quality: recommendations for the English NHS system of quality improvement. 2008.
7. World Health Organisation. Quality of care: a process for making strategic choices in health systems. Geneva: World Health Organisation; 2006.
8. Institute of Medicine. Crossing the quality chasm: a new health system for the 21st century. 2001.
9. Mosadeghrad AM. A conceptual framework for quality of care. Mat Soc Med. 2012;4:251–61.
10. Maxwell RJ. Dimensions of quality revisited: from thought to action. Qual Health Care. 1992;1:171–7.
11. Taylor SL, Dy S, Foy R, et al. What context features might be important determinants of the effectiveness of patient safety practice interventions? BMJ Qual Saf. 2011;20:611–7.
12. Pronovost P, Sexton B. Assessing safety culture: guidelines and recommendations. Qual Saf Health Care. 2005;14:231–3.
13. Porter M, Lee T. The strategy that will fix healthcare. Harv Bus Rev. 2013;91(12):24.
14. Lewis R, Edwards N. Improving length of stay: what can hospitals do? London: Nuffield Trust; 2015. www.nuffieldtrust.org.uk.
15. Donabedian A. The quality of care: how can it be assessed? J Am Med Assoc. 1988;260(12):1743–8.
16. Øvretveit J. Health service quality: an introduction to quality methods for health services. Oxford: Blackwell; 1992.
17. Martin GP, McKee L, Dixon Woods M. Beyond metrics? Utlising 'soft intelligence' for healthcare quality and safety. Soc Sci Med. 2015;142:19–26.
18. Manchester Patient Safety Framework. http://www.nrls.npsa.nhs.uk/resources/?entryid45=59796.
19. Mid Staffordshire NHS Foundation Trust. Public inquiry—chaired by Robert Francis QC. Final report. 3 volumes. 2013. www.midstaffspublicinquiry.com/report.
20. http://www.akumen.co.uk/wp-content/resources/measuring_whats_important.pdf

Factors Affecting Failure

2

Ahmed Nassef, Louise Ramsden, Amanda Newnham, Gareth Archer, Robert Jackson, James Davies, and Kay Stewart

At a time of global economic downturn, there is a temptation for healthcare organisations to focus on cost reduction rather than on quality improvement as a business strategy. However such a strategy can indeed be a dangerous one for patients, [1] with recommendations that the best strategy to advance cost savings is to improve the health status of patients through quality improvement [1–4].

However despite evidence for factors contributing to successful global healthcare systems [5] the report into the failings of the UK Mid Staffordshire hospital inquiry outlined *"first and foremost the appalling suffering of many patients. This was primarily caused by a serious failure on the part of the (healthcare) provider Trust Board who did not listen sufficiently to its patients and staff or ensure the correction of deficiencies brought to the Trust's attention"* [6].

The investigation identified a number of factors that contributed to the Mid Staffordshire Hospital's failure (Table 2.1). This chapter will set out each of these factors in turn and draw upon case studies to highlight examples of how quality improvement can play a part in developing a patient focused quality strategy for hospitals.

Successful hospitals have a quality improvement culture, where patient safety is an integral part of how quality is defined [7, 8] and clinical leadership is evident in the way clinicians work in partnership with patients to improve health care [9]. However, in England, UK out of 274 NHS Trusts, only seven have hospital wide quality improvement strategies [10]. One of these hospitals is Sheffield Teaching Hospitals (STH) who have the Microsystems Coaching Academy (MCA) which is an initiative developed within the Institute of Healthcare Improvement [11]. We will be drawing upon three case studies from this hospital in this chapter.

A. Nassef (✉) • J. Davies • K. Stewart
Sheffield Teaching Hospitals NHS Foundation Trust, Sheffield, UK
e-mail: Ahmed.Nassef@sth.nhs.uk; James.davies84@doctors.org.uk; Kay.Stewart@sth.nhs.uk

L. Ramsden
Sheffield Children's NHS Foundation Trust, Sheffield, UK
e-mail: Louise.ramsden@nhs.net

A. Newnham
Alumni Future Leaders Programme, Health Education England: Yorkshire and the Humber, Leeds Children's Hospital NHS Foundation Trust, Leeds, UK
e-mail: Amanda.newnham@nhs.net

G. Archer
Fellow in Cardiology, Sheffield, UK
e-mail: garetharcher@nhs.net

R. Jackson
Harrogate and District NHS Foundation Trust, Harrogate, UK
e-mail: mrrobjackson@gmail.com

P. Godbole et al. (eds.), *Why Hospitals Fail*, DOI 10.1007/978-3-319-56224-7_2

Table 2.1 Factors affecting hospital failure: *Source: letter to the Rt Hon Jeremy Hunt accompanying the report of the Mid Staffordshire NHS Foundation Trust Pubic Enquiry* [6]

	Factors affecting failure	Case study/examples for an alternative scenario
1.	A culture focused on doing the 'system's business' not that of the patient	Case Study 1: Developing a culture of Quality Improvement
2.	An institutional culture which ascribed more weight to positive information about the service rather than information implying concern	Case Study 2: Developing a culture of openness for a 'duty of candour'
3.	Standards and methods of measuring compliance which did not focus on the effect of a service on patients	Case Study 3: End of Life care, engaging with patients families with a bereavement survey
4.	Too great a degree of tolerance of poor standards and of risk to patients	
5.	A failure of communication between agencies to share their knowledge of concern	Case Study 4: Developing effective communication and staff engagement
6.	A failure to tackle challenges to the building up of a positive culture in nursing and medicine	
7.	Assumptions that monitoring, performance management or intervention was the responsibility of someone else	Case Study 5: A need for whole organisation and support with engagement in quality improvement
8.	A failure to appreciate the risk of disruptive loss of corporate memory and focus resulting from repeated multi-level reorganisation	Case Study 6: A case for Medical Leadership to build capability in the organisation to embed quality improvement

2.1 Case Study 1: From a Culture Focused on Doing the 'System's Business' to a Culture of 'Quality Improvement'

The following example of a Quality Improvement Leadership Programme was set up by Health Education England (HEE) across the Yorkshire and the Humber, UK, and led by ANe as she worked as a Leadership Fellow in an 'out of programme' Quality Improvement programme for the period of a year. The project set out to engage, teach and evaluate a Quality Improvement programme for junior doctors.

Health Education England (HEE) across Yorkshire and Humber in the UK is an arms length organisation responsible for overseeing the training of junior doctors and allied healthcare professionals. It is responsible for "ensuring that the health workforce of today has the right numbers, skills, values and behaviours" to deliver "excellent healthcare and health improvement" [12]. The project has chosen to focus on training of junior doctors as they are the "eyes and ears" of the NHS [6] whose energy should be "tapped not sapped" [13] in improving healthcare. Junior doctors are in a unique position as they rotate through organisation and specialties within the region as part of their training and in empowering them to undertake service improvement projects they can share these experiences and learn about leadership in the process [14]. A pilot QI programme was delivered in the East of the region involving four hospitals and focusing on two specialties (core medical and anaesthetic trainees ST1-2). This would encompass a potential of 107 trainees (Table 2.2).

The Introduction to Quality Improvement (QI) course development was based on the limited evidence base available, as despite there being over 5000 article published on QI training of healthcare professionals these are mainly descriptive of the training content rather than focusing on measuring the impact of the assumption that the training will translate into meaningful improvements in patient safety and the quality of care [15]. The evidence showed that practical, not didactic, teaching focused around a "real-life" work based problem is the most effective form of learning [15]. Therefore attendees were asked to bring a problem from their work place to work through as an example

Table 2.2 Trainee post allocation in East Yorkshire

Trainee allocation per NHS Trust	Acute care common stem & anaesthetics	Core medical	Total
Hull & East Yorkshire NHS Trust	6	37	43
Harrogate & District Foundation Trust	2	7	9
Northern Lincolnshire & Goole Foundation Trust (NLAG)	7	18	25
York Teaching Hospital Foundation NHS Trust (includes Scarborough)	7	23	30
			Overall total 107

using the improvement model structure [16] with day one covering tools to define the problem, setting and aim and measurements. The second day was a month later and the expectation was that they would bring their baseline data and learn more about how to analyse it, troubleshoot their project and consider their next PDSA (Plan, Do, Study, Act) cycle. After the course had been delivered, the Academy of Medical Royal Colleges (AoRMC) released national guidance on QI education for healthcare professionals in the "Training for better Outcomes" Report [17] including a curriculum that should be covered; reassuringly the IQI mapped well to this curriculum (Table 2.3).

The course was evaluated for its overall content and knowledge acquirement by attendees using a self-rated paper based evaluation tool of the days of the course. This has been termed a "Reactionnaire" and was important to identify areas of improvement and potential missed topics to allow fine tuning but should not be used as the long term sole evaluation tool [18]. This assessed the first two levels of Kirkpatrick's learning evaluation model [19]. The evaluation demonstrated an overall improvement in knowledge of IQI from 4.4 to 8.2 (scale 1–10) at the end of the course. This aligns with the evidence that training healthcare professionals in QI has the potential to impact positively on attitudes, knowledge and behaviours [20].

The overall pilot project was challenging for several reasons and required an adaptive approach to leadership and consideration of different influencing styles. A lack of an initial stakeholder analysis was problematic; this has been shown to be associated with failure of change initiatives [21]. An enthusiastic adopter method had been used to select the EAST of the region and the specialist schools self-selecting themselves to be part of the pilot. This had led to initial meetings and agreement in principal for the course. However there was significant disparity between the ideas and expectations of the two sides. This highlighted how a task-orientated leadership approach, prior to the author's role, to ensure planning, monitoring and ownership of the project by all stakeholders would have been beneficial [22]. On reflection the project left the author with feelings akin to the "heroic leader" [23] with the focus on the leader driving forward the training course. It was felt a difficult and challenging situation for the author who was a trainee working outside the organisation and who lacked the legitimate power base or authority to exert the required influence within the organisation [24]. Attempts to increase influence and power through the supervisor and through connections to the Director of Medical Education within each organisation were an important part of the change strategy. A relational leadership style would have been beneficial for this project using a distributed leadership model allowing the course and its direction to be co-designed and co-created with the followers [25]. This was difficult to achieve as the management of the programme was considered as a "pilot" and occurred just days before delivery of the first course. The relational approach had not been used by the leadership fellow who had led the project a year previously, which suggests that a focus on implementing a quality improvement project without consideration of a leadership strategy is likely not be effective. The sustaining engagement of trainees in undertaking QI projects over time was likely lost after the training, due to a lack of engagement in this process by the sponsoring organisations. This was evidenced by the QI trainee participants not having access to support, resources or the opportunity for growth and feedback from their projects at their presentation.

In the future, the plan is to undertake a stakeholder analysis and include strategies for patients and public engagement. This will result in

Table 2.3 Introduction to Quality Improvement (IQI) course overview & curriculum alignment

	IQI course	AoMRC curriculum (knowledge)
Day 1: Aims	To understand the basics of QI	
Day 1: Objectives	Understand:- Quality in healthcare What Quality Improvement is What a Quality Improvement project is	**UG**: compare and contrast quality assurance and quality improvement
Day 1: Session content	• Patient story • What is Quality & Quality Improvement • QI Vs Audit • The Improvement model • Activity on prototyping • Tools for defining the problem e.g. process mapping • Surgery to develop QI Project; setting aims and deciding about measurements	**UG**: QI in clinical governance Describe PDSA cycles Understand difference in principle is QI/research/audit **CT**: Describes tools available for planning quality improvement interventions. Explains process mapping, goal and aim setting **HT**: Compares and contrasts the principles of measurement for improvement, judgment and research.
Day 2: Aim	To be able to undertake a QI project	**CT**: Designs, implements, completes & evaluates a simple quality improvement project using improvement methodology as part of a multidisciplinary team.
Day 2: Objectives	Understand:- How to use and interpret measures in QI project How to undertake a stakeholder analysis How different leadership styles relate to QI How to influence & engage others in QI projects	**HT**: Describes types of measures, and methods of assessing variation
Day 2: Session Content	• Revision day 1 & Improvement model • Leadership styles, influence & stakeholder analysis • Activity on PDSA cycles • Variation, run charts and SPC charts • Surgery to continue development of QI project.	**CT**: Explains stakeholder analysis, statistical methods of assessing variation, implementing change.

AoMRC curriculum key: *UG* undergraduate, *FT* Foundation training, *CT* Core/basic training, *HT* Higher training

inverting the structure of the course so that it is delivered and ran locally to aid engagement and move towards being supported by a relational leadership style. It is hoped that such an approach will result in co-production and a greater ownership of quality improvement across the medical specialties. This has emphasised the importance of co-designing processes for measuring the impact of training outcomes of a training course from the outset of the project, as opposed to being an ad hoc approach. However further work needs to be undertaken to assess the impact of the improvement projects on the patient experience.

2.2 Case Study 2: Developing a Culture of Openness Though a 'Duty of Candour'

A statutory duty of candour was introduced for health and social care as a recommendation of the failings of the Mid Staffordshire Hospital inquiry

(Francis 2013). This was defined by Sir Robert Francis in the following way:

Openness—enabling concerns and complaints to be raised freely without fear and questions asked to be answered.

Transparency—allowing information about the truth about performance and outcomes to be shared with staff, patients, the public and regulators.

Candour—any patient harmed by the provision of a healthcare service is informed of the fact and an appropriate remedy offered, regardless of whether a complaint has been made or a question asked about it.

It is the focus on Candour that we will now explore and identify the impact and barriers of this statutory requirement. Since the inquiry [6] English Health and Social Care Services Regulator, the Care Quality Commission (CQC) registration requirements are that NHS Trusts should write to notify a patient (or their representative) of any incident from which death, moderate or severe physical harm, or prolonged psychological harm has resulted. The notification should include an apology, details of the incident and details of any enquiry into the incident. Reasonable support should also be offered to the patient [26].

The CQC requirement follows in the path of initiatives including the 'Being Open' framework from the NHS National Patient Safety Agency, United States America (USA) [27]. The requirement for healthcare professionals to be open and honest about clinical incidents is included in the General Medical Council (GMC) 'Good Medical Practice' [28], and the Nursing and Midwifery Council (NMC) code of standards [29]. A candid approach is also advocated by indemnity bodies including the Medical Protection Society (MPS) and Medical Defence Union (MDU) [30].

When considering the implementation of the duty of candour, it is important to consider whether the implementation of such a policy would affect the rates of incident reporting. The ability of NHS risk management departments to evaluate and respond to risks is dependent upon clinical incident and 'near miss' reports being generated by front-line staff. It is also important to consider what the barriers to disclosure of clinical incidents to patients are and whether the duty of candour is likely to influence these.

Within the consultation period for the duty of candour, a consultation document by the Royal College of Surgeons considered the impact of the duty of candour upon 'Safety and Improvement'. The authors proposed that "*By being honest with patients and carers, providers of care are far more likely to be honest with themselves*" ([30], p. 12). They argued that by building a culture of honesty, healthcare organisations will be able to learn from their errors and use this as the basis for improvement and harm reduction.

Dalton and Williams [30] reflected that the number of clinical incidents reported through the UK National Reporting and Learning Service (NRLS) did not represent the true number that are believed to occur, when compared to estimates gained from retrospective case reviews. The authors argued that it would be necessary to cause a major change in culture regarding candour and disclosure in order to produce a significant change to error reporting practice. The authors suggest that the duty of candour will be a catalyst for this change, though its implementation will require time and money to be dedicated to staff education and training.

A counter argument is expressed in part of the Department of Health impact assessment [31] who cite unattributed representations from healthcare providers and professionals suggesting that fear of litigation may cause providers to avoid initiating candid conversations with patients. Paradoxically, this would risk the implementation of the duty of candour leading to the promotion of a culture of secrecy.

The principle of using a top-down approach of legislation and policy to affect behaviour change for incident and error reporting in the UK is one which does not have a substantial evidence base. There is no direct evidence available to demonstrate that the 'Being Open' framework [27] has influenced incident reporting behaviour.

US authors have commented that historically there had been a professional culture of discretion and cover-up following medical incidents and errors [32, 33]. However, a number of regulatory and legislative changes have occurred in recent years. The USA 'Joint Commission' is a not-for-profit healthcare inspector and accreditor which has parallels to the CQC in the UK (although other accreditation boards are available). Its 2007 requirements for accreditation of healthcare organisations stated that "*Patients... are informed about the outcomes of care and services that have been provided, including unanticipated outcomes*" [34].

Attempts to legislate for disclosure at a federal level, such as the Clinton and Obama 'Medical Error Disclosure and Compensation' (MEDIC) bill of 2005, have failed to pass through congress. However, nine individual states have passed legislation requiring healthcare providers to inform patients of 'serious events' or 'unanticipated outcomes' [32, 34]. A number of other states have introduced 'apology laws', offering legal protection from malpractice claims to physicians when they make an apology. However, this protection does not usually extend to any further explanation or admission of negligence [34].

Again, there is no direct evidence from the USA to show that the rate of incident reporting has improved with the implementation of this legislation. There is, however, indirect evidence relating to the barriers faced by healthcare professionals when discussing clinical incidents with patients and the attitudes of healthcare professionals towards disclosure. Perhaps unsurprisingly for USA literature, the majority of the evidence relates to the litigation consequences of disclosure.

2.2.1 Barriers to Disclosure

A range of enabling and impeding factors to medical error reporting by physicians were identified by Kaldjian et al. [35]. These factors were arranged into four thematic groups; attitudes, fears, uncertainties and feelings of helplessness. This provides a system for categorising barriers identified by other studies. Kaldjian et al. [35] did not specifically examine the issue of disclosure of errors to patients, but several of the factors identified are relevant to the implementation of duty of candour.

Attitudinal barriers identified included perfectionism, arrogance, and self interest. These were supported by evidence from Garbutt et al. [36] who studied the attitudes of paediatricians towards disclosure of serious incidents. Factors which would deter disclosure included the belief that the patient's family would not understand the explanation, or that they would not want to know, demonstrating the influence of arrogant and paternalistic attitudes. Waring [37] interviewed UK physicians and identified an attitude which rejected 'outside influences', particularly those of 'management' and 'bureaucracy', resulting in a reduced tendency to report errors.

Uncertainties were also seen as barriers, in particular uncertainty about which errors to disclose, and how to disclose them. Singh et al. [38] surveyed healthcare professionals working in the University of Tennessee Hospital, Chattanooga. They identified that only 68% of physicians and 48% of non-physicians were aware that disclosure was recommended, highlighting a deficit in education and training within their organisation and a lack of clear protocols and guidelines. Lack of certainty on what constituted an error, difficulties in identifying when errors occurred and uncertainty over whose responsibility it was to disclose the error were all identified in a study of disclosure practice in the out of hospital (or prehospital in UK terminology) setting by Lu et al. [33]. Interestingly, Garbutt et al. [36] showed that paediatricians might not disclose information if they thought that the patient's family were unaware that an error had occurred, demonstrating a fundamental lack of understanding of the principle of disclosure.

Fear of litigation, damage to professional reputation and to career prospects, and fear of a breakdown of the patient-professional relationship were also barriers to disclosure. Fear of litigation was consistent to all studies, including those of UK doctors [37]. Garbutt et al. [36] specifically cite the fear that a patient's family might become angry following disclosure as a barrier in the paediatric setting.

Finally, feelings of helplessness produced barriers to disclosure. Examples included the impressions that disclosing errors penalises those who are honest, and that by disclosing errors clinicians 'lose control' of the situation [35]. Other practical concerns were identified including the feeling that clinicians lacked the time to make disclosures, or had difficulty making disclosures once care of a patient had passed to a different clinical team [33]. Garbutt et al. [36] found that clinicians found it difficult to disclose information to patients they did not feel they knew well enough.

Perhaps reassuringly, enabling factors for disclosure by physicians included the feeling of responsibility towards the patient, themselves, their profession, and society; i.e. to be honest and respectful to the patient, to be accountable for their own actions, and to maintain trust within the profession [35]. 97% of paediatricians surveyed supported disclosure of serious events to patients and their families [36].

In a culture in which patients expect greater autonomy and in which there is less deference for medical and healthcare professionals, it is necessary for open disclosure to patients of clinical incidents and errors to occur. This has been recognised and acted on by a number of organisations in UK healthcare as mentioned previously. The evidence, however, shows that there are many other barriers that prevent healthcare professionals from disclosing such incidents to patients. It would therefore seem rational that these issues should be addressed within a Quality Improvement programme in order to ensure that implementation of the policy is successful.

2.3 Case Study 3: Engaging Patients and Their Carers in the Development of Best Practice in 'End of Life Care'

How health organisations care for dying people is a critical topic in health care. It is important to both the general public and to health care workers. More recently, it has been at the forefront of issues raised by the Francis Inquiry into Mid Staffordshire NHS trust (Francis 2013), which heard *"Privacy and dignity, even in death, were denied"* in too many instances. It goes to the heart of the criticisms regarding use and abuse of the Liverpool Care Pathway for the Care of the Dying [39] that were investigated by Baroness Julia Neuberger [40] in the UK. The Liverpool Care Pathway had been recommended practice in caring for dying people since the NHS End-of-Life Care strategy 2008 suggested rolling it out nationally [41]. Neuberger et al. [40] *"found repeated instances of patients dying on the LCP being treated with less than the respect that they deserve"* [40]. One of the primary recommendations was that the Liverpool Care Pathway was withdrawn from use.

Following on from Francis and Neuberger there was a move to re-evaluate how dying people are cared for, and also how organisations are inspected on the care that they give. There were two key developments to come out of this. The Leadership Alliance for the Care of Dying People (LACDP) was formed, which was made up from 21 national organisations, and was tasked with responding to the recommendations from the Neuberger Review. They published a document in June 2014 which set out the recommended approach for individuals and for organisations in caring for the dying. "One Chance to Get it Right" [42] gave five priorities for care that individuals and organisations should endeavor to achieve. The Care Quality Commission (CQC), with a new focus on acute hospitals [26], now inspect eight core themes, with end-of-life care as one of these.

The imperative then is for organisations to provide a quality service in caring for those at the end of their life. This creates a dilemma in that there are aspects of palliative and end-of-life care that are difficult to measure. The concept of a "good death" refers to more than just adequately treated symptoms, but to the many other dimensions of the experience.

2.3.1 Relatives as Proxies

As death is not always predictable, so studying people's experiences prospectively is not always possible, using bereaved relatives as a proxy for the person who died has long been used in research. The seminal work in *Life before Death*

[43] interviewed bereaved families to describe the experiences of adults in their last year of life. The authors interviewed both patients and their relatives, but at different time points and about different aspects of their care, making it hard to correlate the views, and raising the question as to how well the bereaved relative reflects the experience of the dying person. This is what validity means here—the proxy's agreement with the patient. Symptoms and other aspects of care can be given a score, and statistical tests used to assess how closely they match.

The other important aspect to this is that bereaved relatives experiences are important in their own right. Part of the care of the dying person is care of the carers, so we are not only interested in their view if it matches the patient's view. Accepting this, it is still important to know whether their view can be said to be a representation of the patient's experience.

There is an ethical and moral implication, in that if bereaved relatives are going to have their grief intruded, there needs to be evidence that it is usable and useful information.

The concept of bereaved relatives as proxies and the potential pitfalls is also acknowledged by researchers in Iran [44], Japan [45] and Korea. They further confirm the importance of this source of information when evaluating how people and organisations care for dying people.

There is evidence then that bereaved relatives can be a useful indicator of quality, but it is important to be cautious in the interpretation. There will always be a need for services to monitor their quality and patient feedback is a major part of the national drive to continuously improve quality.

In the USA there was work done to develop a tool-kit of measurement tools to capture patient and family perspectives in end-of-life care (TIME). Teno et al. ([46, 47]) developed a retrospective bereavement survey by interviewing six focus groups of bereaved relatives, undertaking a qualitative literature review of professional guidelines, and contacted experts for opinion on what constitutes quality care at the end-of-life. From this they "defined five central elements of patient-focussed, family-centred health care". A survey to measure this from the family's perspective was developed. There was an effort to base the survey on a conceptualisation of a good death as defined by professional opinion, professional guidelines and interviews with bereaved relatives, however the guidelines and opinion obtained are heavily focussed on the United States with little international or UK opinion. This is relevant as the concept of a good death differs from person to person, and has major politico-socio-cultural influences. Furthermore, the people recruited for the focus groups were not representative of the wider population in that there were few from minority ethnic backgrounds and were from only a few areas of the US.

In Japan, Morita et al. [45] used satisfaction as the basis for their "scale to measure satisfaction of bereaved family receiving inpatient palliative care". Using a combination of an expert panel and a review of the literature on satisfaction in healthcare the scale was developed. They were able to show validity and reliability of their tool, but when it was used the results showed significant skewing towards satisfaction over dissatisfaction. This is significant, because if the tool fails to pick up aspects of care that could be improved then it is not helpful in the context of quality improvement.

In the United Kingdom the Views of Informal Carers for the Evaluation of Services (VOICES) survey has been developed. It has progressed from work done in the 1990s [48] auditing deaths and experiences of people dying from cancer, based on previous work done by Cartwright et al. [43]. Following this a randomised controlled trial conducted by Addington-Hall et al. [49] was undertaken. Here it was established that using a postal method did not give significantly different results to a face to face interview (although it was noted that face to face interviews did lead to more positive responses, more data was missing in postal responses and the answers were less reliable). The VOICES survey itself was created for the RCT, using expert opinion of palliative care specialists, GP's, nurses and by use of piloting with bereaved relatives. This tool was subsequently used across multiple settings both in and out of hospital.

VOICES has now been used in a variety of settings and clinical conditions and has become part of Department of Health policy. The end of life care strategy recommends rolling VOICES programmes out [41].

The use of bereaved relatives as a proxy for the experience of a dying person is not without problems, but it is an established method of collecting information with evidence that the data gathered is reliable. There are a wide variety of bereavement tools that have been developed in different healthcare settings and countries making use of bereaved relative's views. Establishing a bereavement survey would be one useful mechanism for an organisation to monitor their success in meeting the priorities for care for dying people that we are now mandated to achieve. More can be done to learn from others worldwide, as to how to engage with patients from across a particular clinical specialty. Our work at Sheffield Teaching Hospitals NHS Trust, UK was carefully developed after a review of the global literature to understand how best to engage with patients and their carers on the end of life pathway. We recommend that this is used to develop a standard to support and inform the engagement of patients and carers in the development of new protocols and guidance in all aspects of clinical practice.

2.4 Case Study 4: Developing an Engaged Workforce to Foster Positive Collaborative Communication

'Engaged staff think and act in a positive way about the work they do, the people they work with and the organisation that they work in' [50]. The more engaged staff members are, the better the outcomes are for patients and the organisation generally [51]. Generating a staff engagement strategy is essential to support a leadership strategy for the organisation as leadership is the most influential factor in shaping organisational culture and so ensuring the necessary leadership behaviours, strategies and qualities are developed is fundamental [52]. The leadership task for hospitals is to protect from failure, is to ensure there is direction, alignment and commitment within teams and organisations [53] within the organisation and external to it.

Robinson and Hayday [54] states there is a crucial role of the manager in facilitating engagement in a study conducted in seven organisations. Effective line management, good two-way communication, effective internal co-operation and a focus on developing staff are all required if staff engagement is to be achieved. However it is important to remember engagement means attaining a strengthened contribution from all, rather than a potentially isolated few managers and leaders.

The core values of the English NHS is to offer safe quality services to people in the community. If there is to be satisfactory engagement of the workforce to deliver services in line with these values, organisational values have an enormous role to play in influencing the debate on choices, beliefs and behaviours of employees [55].

Research suggests doctors have the most influence when it comes to implementing operational changes that can lead to improved performance [55]. As it is the people in the organisation who influence the culture of an organisation, the culture in healthcare can be defined as the clinician's perception of events, practices and procedures and should reflect the kinds of behaviour that gets rewarded, supported and expected by the organisation [56].

An organisation's culture needs to support behaviours that enable clinical engagement as effective peer relationships lead to highly engaged, productive employees and drives up organisation performance and improved patient outcomes. There is also a need to support the positive communication between doctors and managers, where managers can support and enable effective medical engagement.

Brooks [57] used the following cultural web to understand some differences in manager and doctor cultures and from an organisational point of view it is necessary to understand the differences in culture in order to arrive at a shared vision:

	Doctors	Managers
Symbols	Stethoscope, stereotypical attire for speciality, titles, colleges, terminology	Reserved parking, dark suits, language/ jargon, laptops
Power structures	Negotiating committees, cliques of 'political' doctors	Executive management team
Control systems	Who knows who, audit	Financial/activity reporting, targets
Rituals and routines	Patient consultations, merit awards	Board meetings, long hours in the office, meetings and committees
Stories	'Us and them', heroes, mavericks, 'in the old days'	'Us and them', things have to change, change is for the best
Paradigm	NHS, a 'good thing', should be free at point of delivery, desire to be the best	NHS, a 'good thing', should be free at point of delivery, desireto be the best

Brooks [57]

The importance of two way communication in engagement has been recognised for years. Kahn [58] found that in an open environment—one in which information was shared freely among organizational members without fear and where meaningful communicative interactions occurred frequently—people were more willing to put all of themselves into their work. If groundwork for meaningful communication is missing, employees' willingness to exert discretionary effort will be missing. Communication is the "lifeblood" of the modern corporation [59].

Research carried out by Institute for Employment Studies (IES) [60] identified that the key driver of employee engagement in the NHS is a sense of feeling valued by, and involved in, the organisation. Staff engagement in the NHS will occur when individuals feel valued and involved. For this, feedback is required and clinicians particularly junior doctors often fail to receive this.

Employers need to provide employees with meaningful career paths, that will inspire and provide them with a variety of opportunities to grow and develop and lead to their goals which will result in greater engagement [60].

A quality improvement project collected data between May and July 2016 [77]. Eleven Trusts in the North of England, UK were sampled. Links to an electronic questionnaire were emailed to all medical staff from distribution lists held either by medical staffing departments or medical education centres, 584 doctors participated. The aim was learn about their experiences in completing incident reports, why they may not be engaged in the process and how this can be improved.

Demographics of grade and speciality were obtained. The percentage of doctors at each grade and specialty completing the questionnaire was compared to their percentage make-up of the total workforce and was used as a surrogate of how engaged participants were with the concept of incident reporting. To measure reporting practice staff were asked how many incidents they had been involved with and how many incident reports they completed within the last year. To determine which factors affected incident reporting 14 factors influencing reporting behaviours were identified and given to participants as options to select from. They were then asked to state what they felt was the most important issue that influenced them completing incident forms. Participants were also encouraged to report any issues and suggestions in free-text comments boxes.

Results showed that clinicians are poor at completing incident report forms; there are a number of factors contributing to this. It was felt that lack of engagement particularly from junior medical staff was a significant factor. This is consistent with other studies [8, 61]. Attitudes and engagement appears to be variable across specialties.

38.2% of doctors felt that not receiving feedback on the forms completed contributed to a lack of engagement in and motivation to filling in incident reports and if feedback was received 425 (73.2%) said they would be more inclined to complete them. The study suggests communication of feedback could and should be improved to improve engagement. Possible solutions were put forward and organisations need to explore ways to listen to its frontline staff if they are to achieve higher levels of staff engagement and in particular medical engagement.

While many of the doctors worked across organisations, it was felt that the forms that organisations required clinicians to complete were of variable standard and there was no agreed standard between organisations. If clinicians were more involved in the design of the forms used this would encourage ownership of the project and hopefully lead to more engagement in the process and better communication across organisations.

With 12.9% of doctors reporting that a fear of repercussions contributes to a poor reporting culture, more needs to be done to engage doctors collectively with managers in designing systems for reporting. While the goal of collective leadership is the engagement of all staff it is important to consider the specific issues that enable the engagement of doctors if we are to change the culture of healthcare. There are obviously still some cultural issues within the NHS despite previous advice to change [6, 8] and these urgently need to be addressed.

2.5 Case Study 5: A Need for Whole Organisation Support with the Engagement of Quality

Batalden and Davidoff [62] defined quality improvement as 'The combined and unceasing efforts of everyone … to make the changes that will lead to better patient outcomes (health), better system performance (care) and better professional development'. However it is the lack of 'collective' responsibility for quality improvement that continues to threaten the continued drive to advance quality in healthcare. This case study outlines a collaborative quality improvement project led by a medical leadership fellow and supported by members of a quality improvement team.

As outlined by the NHS Institute for Innovation and Improvement (Boaden et al. 2008), there are several different methods that can be used to assist quality improvement across healthcare. These include the Plan Do Study Act (PDSA) cycle, Statistical Process Control, Lean, Six Sigma and the Theory of Constraints to name a few. Perhaps key to success is the utilisation of a structured approach to quality improvement with strong and effective leadership, rather than reliance on any one specific method used. However the use of data to inform process improvement through PDSA cycles is essential.

Sheffield Teaching Hospitals NHS Foundation Trust, UK has developed the Microsystems Coaching Academy (MCA) in partnership with the Dartmouth Institute Microsystem Academy (USA). The MCA define microsystems as the 'building blocks of the health care system' and 'the small functional frontline units that provide most health care to most people'. Their approach to quality improvement is to engage those working within a clinical microsystem in 'a structured process to improve the quality of care for patients and the staff who work there'. Improvement in healthcare is more likely to be successful when led by clinicians rather than managers [4], therefore drawing on the expertise of clinical staff and an enthusiasm to deliver quality care helps to initiate change.

One such project was initiated by clinicians on the Acute Medical Unit who wished to obtain data about the doctor processing time of new patient admissions and formally identify suspected systems inefficiencies within the process. This was in light of rising hospital admissions, winter bed pressures, increasing concerns regarding the availability of medical staffing, and the ability of the hospital to cope with this paradox. The ideal hospital admissions process is efficient and predictable with minimal variation between patients. However, medical patients can be complex with a variety of presenting conditions and therefore a degree of variation in processing time is inevitable. Removing as many system inefficiencies as possible will create a timely and efficient admissions process, which will reduce variation within the system and thereby increase predictability. This, in turn, will reduce the need for a variable capacity which can be very difficult to manage, particularly within the confines of definitive bed and staffing numbers.

The data required to assess the process of medical admissions was obtained by a multi-professional team shadowing junior doctor shifts, and recording activity and duration. The data collection team comprised of four team members with a variety of managerial and quality improvement backgrounds, and was led by a clinician (LR) working as a Leadership Fellow. The data obtained confirmed the key activities undertaken by the junior doctors and allowed calculation of the time spent with each patient. This also allowed repetitive or menial tasks to be identified and highlighted as opportunities for change.

This data demonstrated that each complete patient episode took much longer than predicted with a mean of 90 min spent completing all tasks relating to a single patient. Perhaps surprisingly, only one third of this time was spent directly with the patient. A large proportion of the remaining time was spent writing notes and ensuring accurate documentation of clinical events. This is a potential reflection of the medico-legal culture which is having an ever increasing influence on medical practice. There was also a reasonable proportion of time wasted on duplicate activities, walking between departments, looking for equipment and repeatedly checking for blood test results. A number of suggestions have subsequently been made to reduce the time spent on these surplus activities such as dedicated quiet desk space for use by medics, and the use of electronic tracking of investigation results. The general process of acute assessment is currently undergoing a Hospital wide review.

Blom and Alvesson [63] describe that typically leadership involves 'influence' as opposed to 'the use of brute force or formal authority' within management or managerial work. The ability to inspire others influences 'followers by providing a moral example or being a role model'. Dazi [9] reported that 'it is important for clinicians to be involved in both informing and leading change'. The importance of strong clinical leadership is well recognised, with Dickinson et al. [64] reporting that better performing trusts have higher levels of clinician engagement. This quality improvement project is a real demonstration of the benefits of putting this academic theory into practice. To have a clinician leading this project was particularly advantageous due to their understanding of the system and practical knowledge about the process of hospital admission. This essential knowledge created a greater power to influence organisational change as well as an ability to inspire a shared purpose in the team, resulting in collective leadership.

2.6 Case Study 6: Medical Leadership as a Mechanism to Build Organisational Capability and a New 'Quality Improvement' Organisational Culture

The most significant leadership of any one particular professional group, (that if absent will cause hospitals to fail), is that of medical leadership. While there is evidence that stable and longevity of chief executive leadership is important [65] for a hospital, there appears to be a lack of attention as to how the organisation can secure more stability and continuity in medical leadership across the hospital Trust. Bohmer [66] outlines that there are two core rationales for medical leadership: (1) the first being a need for doctors to keep politicians focussed on the design of health structures and funding mechanisms. His argument is that whatever the politicians do they cannot do this without the involvement of doctors and (2) doctors are involved in the intimate day to day practice with optimal organisational knowledge in delivery of clinical practice. Medical leadership has been attributed to improved operational performance "improvements happen because clinicians most notably doctors played an integral part in shaping clinical services" [5, 66, 67]. In addition there is evidence that doctors are closest to the evidence based practice that informs protocols and guidance which in turn inform team or clinical microsystems. In conclusion Spurgeon summarises evidence to show that "organisations in which doctors are engaged in maintaining and enhancing the performance of the organisation, perform better financially and clinically" [68]. There is now a generally accepted view that medically led services are "when the doctor is taking a leadership role in the doing" [69] which should be the vision for future healthcare.

However the context of healthcare continues to be challenging, with increased demands on healthcare with a worldwide aging population as well as complex care needs and rising costs of care [66]. Organisational restructuring of healthcare in the UK with Clinical Commissioning Groups has placed an increased demand for the skills of medical leadership across the hospital and community sector. While demand for medical leadership is rising, at the same time there are increases in the volume of clinical episodes, while patients themselves expect greater value in the patient–doctor relationship.

As the demand for medical leadership has increased "doctors have become demonstrably disengaged from the systems of which they are a key part" [66]. Reasons for this could be down to (1) Doctors are becoming disengaged because of a drive towards targets and not quality performance or (2) the management of health services are increasing in complexity and doctors may not have the skills or knowledge or time to address this. Studies have been undertaken to examine medical engagement and strategies to overcome them, but while some interventions such as leadership programmes have been introduced, the problem is still a global problem with very little evidence that medical leadership programmes are achieving greater medical engagement that results in improved organisational performance [68]. The few studies of physician leadership that documented favourable organisational outcomes such as improvements in quality indicators were characterised by the use of multiple learning methods and involved action learning and projects in multi-disciplinary teams [70].

This case study illustrates how a medical leadership programme can be embedded in a hospital, by using processes of co-design and co-production with medical leaders, to engage doctors in creating a medical leadership programme that is 'fit for purpose' and will support their clinical practice. The programme specification was produced as a result of the consultation process undertaken with Clinical Leads (CL), Clinical Directors (CD) and other senior stakeholders at Sheffield Teaching Hospital NHS Trust, UK. The specification also built upon, and supported, the vision of the Chief Executive Officer, Sir Andrew Cash, which was shared with senior clinical leaders at a Leadership event.

The broad strategy of the CLs Leadership Development Programme was to build on this vision for medical leadership to:

- Engage all Clinical Leads in the co-design of a bespoke medical leadership development programme.
- Identify the leadership development needs of individual Clinical Leads and plan a curriculum to best meet these needs.
- Identify with each Clinical Lead a service improvement project to act as the vehicle for their leadership learning and development.
- Draw on and use multiple data sets, e.g., patients, financial, etc. and then subsequently apply appropriate statistics tools to present a baseline of the problem.
- Support the programme with individual leadership development diagnostics, jointly agreed with STH Learning and Development Centre, to generate leadership diagnostic data for the dual purpose of (1) providing feedback on individual participants' leadership development and (2) generating data for evaluation of the impact of the programme.

A steering group was convened to oversee the development of the curriculum design and manage the implementation of the programme and a subcommittee emerged and was specifically tasked to:

- Undertake one to one interviews with Clinical Leads
- Undertake a 'gap analysis' of the presenting needs of CLs and create a bespoke curriculum to meet their needs
- outline the underlying programme theory;
- set out the learning objectives and outcomes;
- present a summary of programme content;
- outline the teaching and learning strategies;
- identify the delivery team
- outline the method of evaluation

The aim of the programme was to generate a Clinical Leads leadership collective, to support the development of tacit and explicit knowledge in leadership and quality/service improvement. It was envisaged that the group's learning was to be facilitated through seamless collaboration with the hospital's Quality Improvement Microsystems Academy. It was anticipated that by the end of the Programme, CLs will be able to:

1. Explain what leadership behaviours and leadership styles have been used to lead a service improvement project, to achieve specific project outcomes
2. Identify specific strategies to drive patient centred quality improvement projects
3. Utilise leadership data and project data to inform future leadership learning
4. Develop specific skills and knowledge in leadership and quality improvement theories and methods
5. Explain the Clinical Leadership role as a form of 'hybrid leadership' to help redefine professional identities
6. Develop situated and distributed leadership behaviours through a reflective frame of the identity of a Clinical Lead role

The outcomes of the programme was the production of eight 'medical leadership and quality improvement' project reports, which evidenced new quality improvement and medical leadership skills and advances in quality and organisational performance.

Specialty/Project	Report title
1. Acute Medicine	A diversion strategy for Acute Medicine in A&E
2. Laboratory Medicine	Developing standardisation in diagnostic testing
3. Emergency Medicine	The development of a strategy for Emergency Medicine
4. Paediatric Dentistry	A strategy to reduce the 18 week wait
5. Palliative Care	The development of team working in palliative care services
6. Ophthalmology	The development of a CPD strategy for a nurse led eye emergency service
7. Laboratory Services	A review of capacity and demand
8. Neurosurgery	A practical guide to 'job planning' for consultants with the alignment of a 'user friendly' directorate plan

A content analysis of the reports showed seven out of eight projects aimed to increase activity at the hospital. However all the seven projects were aiming to achieve this over the longer term (12–18 months) and none of them would achieve increased measurable activity within a 6 month period. Project 2 sought to decrease activity (in diagnostic testing) where this was not clinically relevant and a waste of resources. This project released time for improvement work in other areas and also demonstrated the project author's authoritative leadership in gathering a consensus from across clinical specialties.

Project 1 increased output/activity if the scheduling of Medically Acute Patients were in a room that was of a sufficiently large size and close to A&E and MAU. There is a direct correlation with the management of space 'ergonomics' and the high volume/throughput in acutely ill medical patients. To enable the sustained embedding of medical leadership in the organisation over time, devolved decision making must be given to these newly 'advanced' skilled clinicians, for them to drive their quality improvement forward. A sense of ownership and responsibility is likely to result in the continued motivation to lead, if clinicians have devolved responsibility. However such devolved responsibility needs to be undertaken within allocated time in the clinician's job work plan.

Project 3 developed a strategy for emergency medicine to increase activity and to prevent breaches to the 4 hours target in A&E. The strategy is multi-layered and has been written to show the complexity between

- Self (awareness of strengths and limitations of individual team members)
- Team (devolving lead roles to members in the team to advance elements of the strategy in relation to the individual strengths of team

members) Team development and team building events

- Organisation (the development of systems for effective planning, control and delivery) systems planning
- Service improvement (the devolvement of quality improvement personnel in Emergency Medicine)

Project 4 initiated a service improvement project in Paediatric dentistry to increase output to manage the waiting list for new patients and the back log. The Clinical Lead has learnt new skills in statistical analysis and for gains to be made (from statistical forecasting) there needs to be a 'systems change' that involves all clinical and non-clinical team members to plan, schedule and deliver the work differently.

Four projects looked specifically at the relationship between commissioned work for clinicians and the capacity of the team to deliver this work. Project 8 developed a strategic 'route map' of the relationship between job planning for clinicians and the commissioned activity from the Directorate and developed a 'user friendly' 'route map' and guide for job planning. This tool needs an implementation group to test out and research the utility of this approach, to identify how such a tool could support greater flexibility in job planning. It is hoped that through the use of this tool that clinicians will be able to identify the relationship between capacity, demand and activity.

Project 5 developed along a similar theme, however the speciality of palliative care presented significant challenges of 'emotional labour'. Staff sickness was significantly higher than other specialties (and higher than the national average) and there were specific challenges of working with patients and their families when patients are in their last hours, days and months of life. The Clinical Lead researched the concept of annualised job planning and worked with the team to develop a shared responsibility to cover the rota to deliver all aspects of the commissioned work. With the support of the team, the clinical lead has managed to influence the rota to halt the sharp rise in sickness levels in this speciality and has created some stability in the team. This has not only saved the Trust money but has created a sustainable infrastructure to reintroduce thinking around quality improvement. A culture of Quality Improvement can only be fostered in a culture of stability for staff and staff wellness. Quality Improvement activity had levelled to a point prior to the high levels of staff sickness.

Project 6 was concerned with the lack of sustainability of the emergency eye service, identifying that there was no CPD strategy for nursing and an absence of a strategy to drive up quality standards in this area. The clinical lead has consulted with the consultant workforce to develop a sustainable infrastructure by engaging consultants in a CPD programme for nurses that will link directly to a governance structure. This was also the focus for project 7 whose medical leader identified high levels of attrition of consultant hours yet the demand for specialist consultant advisory services from the Clinical Commissioning Group (CCG) was increasing. By undertaking an analysis of the demand, capacity and activity, the doctor has generated data for workforce planning and the allocation of work to various grades of staff with the required skill mix.

Embedding medical leadership programmes through a process of co-design and co-production is the way forward to manage the limited time available for medical leadership programmes (this programme was delivered over a half day once a month over 7 months, with tutorials in between). Supporting clinical leaders to produce quality improvement reports is a core element of the programme to evidence outcomes and impact from medical leadership development. However such activity in Quality Improvement can only be undertaken if it is an agreed and scheduled part of a clinician's job work plan.

Acknowledgements We would like to express our thanks and appreciation to the doctors who worked on this programme and who are Dr Ali Cheema, Dr Helena Parkinson, Dr Avril Kuhrt, Ms Halla Zaitoun, Dr Ellie Smith, Dr Irene Pepper, Dr Hannah Delaney and Mr Thomas Carroll.

References

1. Wagner E. Chronic disease management: what will it take to improve care for chronic illness. Eff Clin Pract. 1998;1:2–4.
2. Deming WE. Out of crisis. Cambridge: MIT Press; 1998.
3. Donabedian A. Evaluating the quality of medical care. Milbank Q. 1966;83(4):691–729.
4. Ovretveit J. Do changes to patient – provider relationships improve quality and save money? London: The Health Foundation; 2012.
5. Baker GR. The roles of leaders in high performing health care systems. London: Kings Fund; 2011.
6. Francis R. Report of the Mid Staffordshire NHS Foundation Trust public enquiry: executive summary. [Online]. London: Mid Staffordshire NHS Foundation Trust Public Inquiry; 2013. http://www.midstaffspublicinquiry.com/sites/default/files/report/Executive%20summary.pdf.
7. Berwick D. To err is human: building a safer health system. Washington: Institute of Medicine, National Academy Press; 1999.
8. Berwick D. A promise to learn – a commitment to act, improving the safety of patients in England. National Advisory Group on the Safety of patients in England; 2013.
9. Dazi A. High quality care for all NHS next stage review final report. London: Department of Health; 2008.
10. Ham C, Berwick D, Dixon J. Improving quality in the English NHS: a strategy for action. London: Kings Fund; 2016.
11. IHI. The breakthrough series: IHI's collaborative model for achieving breakthrough improvement. IHI innovation series white paper. Boston: Institute for Healthcare Improvement; 2003. www.IHI.org
12. Health Education England. Health Education England; Our Values. [Online]. 2016. Last updated unknown, accessed 22 May 2016. https://hee.nhs.uk/about-us/our-values.
13. Keogh B. Review into the quality of care and treatment provided by 14 hospital trusts in England: an overview report. Wakefield: NHS England; 2013.
14. Penglington C, Marshall P. Why Junior Doctors are innovation leaders. [Online]. 2013. Last updated 12/0/2013. http://www.hsj.co.uk/topics/leadership/why-junior-doctors-are-innovation-leaders/5060206.fullarticle.
15. The Health Foundation. Encourage, I.I.D. Evidence Scan: quality improvement training for healthcare professionals, 2012.
16. Langley G, et al. The improvement guide: a practical approach to enhancing organizational performance. San Francisco: Jossey Bass Publishers; 1996.
17. Vaux E. Quality improvement - training for better outcomes. London: Academy of Royal Medical Colleges; 2016.
18. Rae L. Assessing the value of your training. The evaluation process from training needs to the report to the board. Aldershot: Gower Publishing Limited; 2002.
19. Kirkpatrick D, Kirkpatrick J. Evaluating training programmes: the four levels. 3rd ed. Oakland: Bereett-Koehler Publishers; 2006.
20. O'Brien MA, et al. Continuing education meetings and workshops: effects on professional practice and health care outcomes. Cochrane Database Syst Rev. 2001;(2).
21. Kotter JP. Leading change: why transformation efforts fail. Harv Bus Rev. 1995;73(2):59–67.
22. West M, et al. Leadership and leadership development in healthcare: the evidence base. London: The Kings Fund; 2015.
23. King's Fund. The future of leadership and management in the NHS: no more heroes. London: The King's Fund; 2011.
24. Pastoriza D, Ariño MA. J Bus Ethics. 2013;118(1). doi:10.1007/s10551-012-1536-7
25. Day D. The Oxford handbook of leadership and organizations. New York: Oxford University Press; 2014.
26. Care Quality Commission. Introducing the statutory duty of candour. [Online]. Leeds: Department of Health; 2014. https://www.gov.uk/government/uploads/system/uploads/attachment_data/file/295773/Duty_of_Candour_Consultation..pdf.
27. National Patient Safety Agency. Being open, [Online]. National Health Service National Patient Safety Agency; 2009. http://www.nrls.npsa.nhs.uk/beingopen/?entryid45=83726.
28. General Medical Council. Good medical practice. [Online]. London: General Medical Council; 2013. http://www.gmc-uk.org/static/documents/content/Good_medical_practice_-_English_0914.pdf.
29. Nursing and Midwifery Council. The code: standards of conduct, performance and ethics for nurses and midwives. [Online]. London: Nursing and Midwifery Council; 2008. http://www.nmc-uk.org/Documents/Standards/The-code-A4-20100406.pdf.
30. Dalton D, Williams N. Building a culture of candour: a review of the threshold for the duty of candour and of the incentives for care organisations to be candid. [Online]. London: Royal College of Surgeons of England; 2014. https://www.rcseng.ac.uk/policy/documents/CandourreviewFinal.pdf.
31. Nolan J, Qian T. Impact assessment: duty of candour on providers. [Online]. London: Department of Health; 2013. https://www.gov.uk/government/uploads/system/uploads/attachment_data/file/295625/DoC_impact-assessment.pdf.
32. Gallagher T, Studdert D, Levinson W. Disclosing harmful medical rrors to patients. [Online]. N Engl J Med. 2007;356(26):2713–9.
33. Lu D, et al. Disclosure of harmful medical errors in out-of-hospital care. [Online]. Ann Emerg Med. 2013;61(2):215–21.
34. Miller L. Apology, disclosure and unanticipated outcomes. [Online]. J Perinat Neonatal Nurs. 2011;25(1):10–1.
35. Kaldjian LC, et al. An empirically derived taxonomy of factors affecting physicians' willingness to disclose

medical errors. [Online]. J Gen Intern Med. 2006;21(9):942–8.
36. Garbutt J, et al. Reporting and disclosing medical errors: pediatricians' attitudes and behaviors. Arch Pediatr Adolesc Med. 2007;161(2):179–85.
37. Waring JJ. Beyond blame: cultural barriers to medical incident reporting. [Online]. Soc Sci Med. 2005;60(9):1927–35.
38. Singh V, et al. Disclosure and documentation of reported unanticipated medical events or outcomes: need for healthcare provider education. [Online]. J Healthc Risk Manag. 2012;32(1):14–22.
39. Mccartney M. The assault on the Liverpool care pathway. [Online]. Br Med J. 2012;345. http://www.bmj.com/content/345/bmj.e7316.
40. Neuberger J, Guthrie C, Aaronvitch D. More care, less pathway: a review of the Liverpool Care Pathway. Department of Health, Crown Copyright; 2013.
41. Great Britain, Department of Health. End of life care strategy: promoting high quality care for all adults at the end of life. [Online]. 2008. https://www.gov.uk/government/uploads/system/uploads/attachment_data/file/136431/End_of_life_strategy.pdf.
42. The Leadership Alliance for the Care of Dying People. Once chance to get it right: improving people's experience of care in the last few days and hours of life. [Online]. 2014. Last updated June 2014. www.gov.uk/government/uploads/system/uploads/attachment_data/file/323188/One_chance_to_get_it_right.pdf.
43. Cartwright A, Anderson J, Hockey L. Life before death. Abingdon: Routledge and Kegan Paul; 1973.
44. Iranmanesh S, Hosseini H, Esmaili M. Evaluating the "good death" concept from Iranian bereaved family members' perspective. J Support Oncol. 2011;9(2):59–63.
45. Morita T, Chihara S, Kashiwagi T. A scale to measure satisfaction of bereaved family receiving inpatient palliative care. Palliat Med. 2002;16(2):141–50.
46. Teno JM, et al. Patient-focused, family-centered end-of-life medical care: views of the guidelines and bereaved family members. J Pain Symptom Manag. 2001;22(3):738–51.
47. Teno JM, et al. Validation of toolkit after-death bereaved family member interview. J Pain Symptom Manag. 2001;22(3):752–8.
48. Addington-Hall J, Mccarthy M. Regional study of care for the dying: methods and sample characteristics. Palliat Med. 1995;9(1):27–35.
49. Addington-Hall J, et al. A randomised controlled trial of postal versus interviewer administration of a questionnaire measuring satisfaction with, and use of, services received in the year before death. J Epidemiol Community Health. 1998;52(12):802–7.
50. The staff engagement toolkit. An online resource, supporting you to increase staff engagement in your organisation. 2013.
51. Dawson J, West M. Summary of key research findings from the NHS staff survey. 2016.
52. Kings Fund. Leadership and leadership development in health care. London: FMLM, Centre for Creative Leadership and Kingsfund; 2015. http://www.kingsfund.org.uk/sites/files/kf/field/field_publication_file/leadership-leadership-development-health-care--feb-2015.pdf.
53. Drath WH, Mccauley CD, Palus CJ, Van Velsor E, O'connor PMG, Mcguire JB. Direction, alignment, commitment: toward a more integrative ontology of leadership. Leadersh Q. 2008;19:635–53.
54. Robinson D, Hayday S. The engaging manager. London: Institute for Employment Studies; 2009.
55. Atkinson S, Spurgeon P, Clark J, Armit K. Engaging doctors: what can we learn from trusts with high levels of medical engagement? London: NHS Institute for Innovation and Improvement and Academy of Medical Royal Colleges; 2011.
56. Schneider B, Ehrhart MG, Macey WH. Organizational climate and culture. Annu Rev Psychol. [Internet]. 2013 Jan 3 [cited 2016 Aug 19];64(1):361–88. Available from: http://www.annualreviews.org/doi/abs/10.1146/annurev-psych-113011-143809.
57. Brooks C. Working with healthcare professionals. Open University Press final report. Healthc Manag. 2006;253–57.
58. Kahn WA. Psychological conditions of personal engagement and disengagement at work. Acad Manag J. 1990;33(334):692–724.
59. Axelrod RH. Terms of engagement: changing the way we change organizations. Oakland: Berrett-Koehler; 2003. p. 240.
60. Robinson D, Perryman S, Hayday S. The drivers of employee engagement. 2004.
61. Hotten E, Jordan L, Pedan C. Improving incident reporting among junior doctors. BMJ Qual Improv Rep. 2014.
62. Batalden PB, Davidoff F. What is "quality improvement" and how can it transform healthcare? Qual Saf Health Care. 2007;16(1):2–3.
63. Blom M, Alvesson M. All-inclusive and all good: the hegemonic ambiguity of leadership. Scand J Manag. 2015;31(4):480–92.
64. Dickinson H, Ham C, Snelling I, Spurgeon P. Are we there yet? Models of medical leadership and their effectiveness: an exploratory study. Southampton: National Institute for Health Research; 2013.
65. IHI (2008) Achieving the vision of excellence in quality: recommendations for the English NHS system of quality improvement. Submitted to the Department of Health by the Institute for Healthcare Improvement. Boston: Institute for Healthcare Improvement.
66. Bohmer R. The instrumental value of medical leadership. London: The Kings Fund; 2012.
67. Mountford J, Webb C. When clinicians lead. McKinsey Q. 2009.
68. Spurgeon P, Long P, Clark J, Daly F. Do we need medical leadership or medical engagement? Leadersh Health Serv. 2015;28(3):173–84.
69. Clark J. Medical leadership and engagement: no longer an optional extra. J Health Organ Manag. [Internet]. [cited 2016 Aug 18] 2012;26(4):437–43.

Available from: http://www.emeraldinsight.com/doi/abs/10.1108/14777261211251517.
70. Frich JC, Brewster AL, Cherlin EJ, Bradley EH. Leadership development programs for physicians: a systematic review. J Gen Intern Med. 2014;30(5):656–74.
71. Addington-Hall J, Mcpherson C. After-death interviews with surrogates/bereaved family members: some issues of validity. J Pain Symptom Manag. 2001;22(3):784–90.
72. Care Quality Commission. New acute hospital inspection model. [Online]. Last updated 19 August 2014. http://www.cqc.org.uk/public/about-us/our-inspections/our-new-acute-hospital-inspection-model.
73. Claessen SJJ, et al. Measuring relatives' perspectives on the quality of palliative care: the consumer quality index palliative care. J Pain Symptom Manag. 2013;45(5):875–84.
74. Department of Health, NHS Medical Directorate. First national VOICES survey of bereaved people: key findings report. Online, Department of Health; 2012.
75. Morita T, et al. Measuring the quality of structure and process in end-of-life care from the bereaved family perspective. J Pain Symptom Manag. 2004;27(6):492–501.
76. Sheffield Microsystems Coaching Academy. Improving a microsystem. [Online]. http://www.sheffieldmca.org.uk/improving_microsystems.
77. Archer, G (2016) A Quality Improvement Project, South Yorkshire and the Humber Deanery (Unpublished).
78. Boaden R (2008) Quality Improvement: Theory and Pratice. British Journal of Healthcare Management Vol15 (1).

3 Assessing the Return on Investment (ROI) Through Appreciative Inquiry (AI) of Hospital Improvement Programmes

Kirtik Patel and Jill Aylott

Across the globe hospitals are struggling financially as they are in a transition to change and support the development of new integrated models of health and social care. The vision and insights of W. Edwards Deming's process management theory argues that the best way to reduce costs is to improve quality. While Deming's principles have been successfully applied in the manufacturing and ser vice sector, it is more challenging to apply these principles to the context of healthcare. Rauh et al (2011) argue that the management and organisation of a typical healthcare setting creates a rigid cost structure that is relativly insensitive to small changes in patient volume, resource use or even in the severity of the patients' health condition. Rauh et al (2011) argue that while fixed costs in healthcare remain relatively unaffected by clinical quality improvements, typically such quality improvements can create additional capacity rat her than bottom line savings. Successful healthcare organisations will create the correct balance between Capacity, Demand and Actvity in order to provide a positive quality experience for patients. This chapter sets out how the metrics to determine a Return on Investment (ROI) calculation can determine the additional capacity that results from a clinical quality improvement project. Due to the complex nature of collective working between a number of stakeholder groups including patients in a hospital setting, it is recommended that dete rmining the ROI should be a collective activity undertaken within a model of Appreciative Inquiry (AI).

While hospitals come under pressure to adapt and change, not all change will result in improvement (or value to the patient) and not all improvement will produce financial returns to the organisation. This chapter will argue that all service improvement programmes should be evaluated using the following questions:

- How much does the patient value this service and how important is this new service rated across the patient's hospital journey?
- To what extent does the new service build in a system to safeguard patient safety?
- What are the returns on investment (ROI) of this improvement or new service?

K. Patel (✉)
Sheffield Teaching Hospitals NHS Trust, Sheffield, UK
e-mail: Kirtik.Patel@sth.nhs.uk

J. Aylott
Directorate for International MBA Programmes, International Academy of Medical Leadership, Sheffield, UK
e-mail: Jill.Aylott@iamedicalleadership.com

P. Godbole et al. (eds.), *Why Hospitals Fail*, DOI 10.1007/978-3-319-56224-7_3

Return on Investment evaluation methodology should be integrated into all change programmes as a key feature to: (1) ensure accountability for the change process of improvement (2) to explore the cost/benefit of any change (3) to increase the confidence of stakeholders in the change process and (4) to provide definitive feedback to the hospital board regarding the percentage of return on investment of a particular change project.

Traditionally quality improvement programmes using Continuous Quality Improvement approaches (e.g. The IHI Breakthrough Series) have implemented rapid change cycles using PDSA (Plan-Do-Study-Act) Breakthrough series (IHI) but such a model is considered by some to inadequately assess the level of risk to the patient. Moving quickly through rapid cycles of change will feel counter-intuitive to doctors who need to be reassured that patients are safe. This is particularly true with the introduction of a nurse led clinic (illustrated in the Case Study for this chapter) where the doctor is ultimately responsible for patients attending the clinic under his or her name. Our case study calls for the use of ROI methodology but within an Action Research framework of Appreciative Inquiry (AI). It is through the mechanism of AI that doctors, nurses, patients and other stakeholders can discuss their particular concerns and issues about 'value' and 'patient safety'. 'Appreciative Inquiry' (AI) is an approach to organisational change which focuses on stengths rather than weaknesses. It has four steps in an interative cycle: Step 1: DISCOVER: experiences, identify strengths and capabilities; Step 2: DREAM: dream and collectively envision what else is possible; Step 3: DESIGN and Step 4: DESTINY (see Fig 3.2). AI enables the recruitment of a key group of people from a range of backgrounds, with patient representation, to come together with specific objectives and to identify how data will be collected, through the AI model. The first author was the facilitator of the AI group alongside the Nurse Specialist. Patient Safety and Value Based Healthcare are are not automatically included in the ROI methodology but are critical to understanding the financial calculation of the ROI in a healthcare context. In our case study there was a ROI of 70.58% which resulted from our clinical quality improvement programme. However this ROI only has significance if patient satisfaction levels remain high and doctors are convinced that patient safety is not compromised.

All service improvement projects are costly and the rationale for a proposal for quality improvement must ultimately be to improve the patient experience and to keep patients safe. All improvement work should engage patients in the process and be firmly established in co-production and the co-creation of new knowledge. With most change projects failing to be sustained over time, a call for a more systematic model to evaluate improvement projects is now required.

Return on investment (ROI) analysis critically evaluates the potential impact of any new service development or quality improvement and also provides comprehensive evaluation data for communicating the impact of the project [1]. Previous economic analysis methodologies within a hospital have required outside consultancy firms and these are costly. The ROI methodology provides a more cost effective and complete picture of costs and of the tangible and intangible benefits to patients and other stakeholders. However it is not intended to be determined by a singular professional/leader. It must be undertaken as a collective activity with all stakeholder groups.

3.1 Return on Investment

Return on Investment (ROI) when used as a financial term, refers in general to the financial return from any financial investment. Within a healthcare organisation this investment may be as a monetary asset, a physical asset (equipment), 'Time' in a Quality Improvement project (leadership program), within a department or in employee performance (learning and development). However, Phillips [2] advocates that a more complete evaluation needs to include both qualitative and quantitative measures. Phillips [2] suggested a Five Level Return on Investment (ROI) Framework. The Five Level Framework adding to a fifth level to Kirkpatrick's [3] four levels of evaluation, with the fifth level

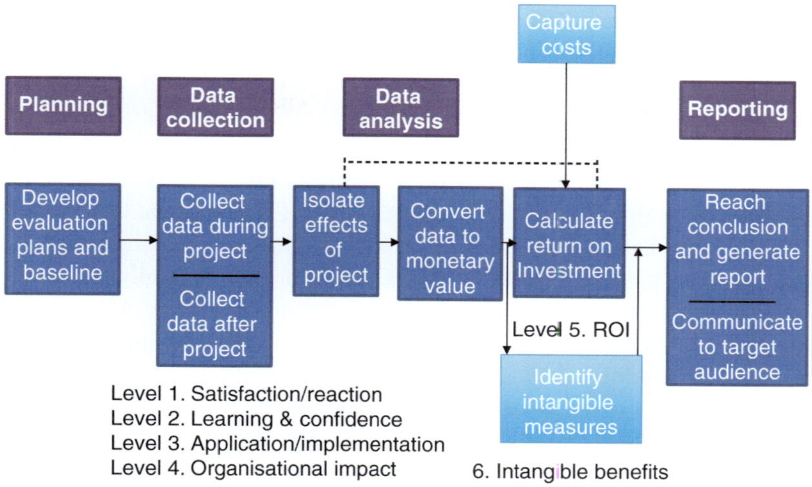

Fig. 3.1 The ROI process model (as taken from Phillips and Phillips)

being the ROI calculation. The ROI process model provides a systematic approach to ROI calculations. The step-by-step approach keeps the process manageable according to Phillips and Phillips [4] and illustrated in Fig. 3.1.

The ROI process model as outlined in Fig. 3.1 is comprehensive in that data metrics are developed at different times from different sources, thus allowing for a more comprehensive evaluation of a project. One of the key steps is the planning stage, where objectives are defined and a planning document agreed. The planning document will include important information concerning the data to be collected, the data sources, the timing of the data collection and the various responsibilities of the group members. The AI group decide how long the group will run for and how often they will meet. There is usually work to be done between each meeting, so setting realistic intervals is important.

The final step in the ROI process is the production of the organisational report. The report is usually presented to the Hospital Board to help communicate how a change project can be undertaken in a systematic way while also being accountable to all stakeholders. It is important to ensure that the report is honest and while reporting the ROI and the process improvements, it will also address some of the 'negative' themes that are raised during the AI process. In our own report there were particular concerns about 'finance' and 'non-recognition by the Trust of the role of the Clinical Nurse Specialist (CNS). The financial viability and the potential to generate income was welcomed by the operational manager and the explicit recording of holistic needs assessments and signposting by the CNS to improve the quality of care for patients was also highly valued by the Nurse Director and Colorectal Matron Practitioner, in effect converting their tacit assumptions into explicit facts.

Our calculations using the ROI method demonstrated that if the pilot was rolled-out and extended over a period of 1 year and assuming that the nurse-led clinic was run on a fortnightly basis for a 40 week service cycle (i.e. 20 clinics) and during each clinic the CNS saw four follow-up patients (in a 2 hour clinic), the income generated would be £6480. This income amounts to more than the cost of covering a CNS Band increment from Band 6 to Band 7. This would hopefully address some of the concerns raised within the AI group about 'non-recognition' by the Trust of the work undertaken by the CNS in relation to the quality of care provided to patients, which requires nurses with advanced levels of training and commitment, as well as the financial and resource implication of employing and retaining CNSs within the Directorate.

The pilot also achieved greater understanding of the value of a nurse-led clinic in helping to signpost patients to appropriate service before a 'crisis' occurs through the holistic needs assessment tool. This could potentially save unnecessary admissions to A&E and inpatient beds or extra clinic appointments to see doctors or GP visits, because problems have been addressed earlier and by empowering patients to seek advice and attempt self-management, because *"it is a journey"* as, stated by an AI group member. The quantification of these additional costs was beyond the scope of this pilot study, however this is highlighted within the NCSI report [5].

The ROI analysis provided an accepted methodology to provide both quantitative and qualitative analysis of the pilot. The financial aspect was particularly relevant to finance managers and the description of the intangible benefits within the report corroborated the tacit knowledge expressed by nursing staff. Action research with the use of AI as a methodology proved to be successful, but an adaption was necessary to allow expression of 'negative' themes. The acknowledgments of these negative themes meant that they could be explored further by the group and potentially be addressed by the pilot study. Nonetheless, the AI process did produce rich narratives and thus facilitated a shared leadership model, which encouraged engagement and empowerment of the various group members.

3.2 A Case Study: Return on Investment for Quality Improvement of a 'Nurse Led' Cancer Follow Up Service

A Quality Improvement project focused on those patients with curative oesophago-gastric cancer resections, and who had received surgery with curative intent and who had no evidence of disease recurrence. Traditionally, doctors and in particular junior doctors, assessing their physical signs and symptoms have undertaken follow-up of these patients. Support is provided from allied healthcare professionals such as the clinical nurse specialist (CNS), dietitians and occasionally physiotherapists.

The introduction of the European Working Time Directive in 2009, limited the number of hours a junior doctor was available for work, which in turn has detrimentally impacted on the number of patients that can be seen in a clinic, thus the majority of patients are now seen by a Consultant [6]. Typically the average time slot available for a routine patient follow-up review has been between 10 and 15 min, thus limiting the amount of time that can be spent assessing each patient, in particular their holistic needs, especially when the number of new patients being referred for a suspected cancer diagnosis is increasing [7].

As a consequence of the need to better serve our cancer follow-up patients and in particular the assessment of their holistic needs, the proposal was for the development of a dedicated CNS led (or clinical nurse specialist -led) cancer follow-up clinic. Although nurse-led clinics are not a new concept [5, 8–10], a ROI had not previously been undertaken to assess the financial value of this service to the organization, while also evaluating the value the service had for patients and assessing the service for risk in relation to patient safety. An AI group was convened Fig. 3.2:

In order to conduct the ROI analysis, one of the first steps was to develop comprehensive evaluation plans and decide on benchmark data metrics for the study. The action group utilised appreciative inquiry (AI) to determine which data to collect and the level of evaluation necessary for the ROI analysis as well as the method of data collection. The group then reconvened again during the data analysis process to determine important confounding factors and also agreed on the calculations to be used to convert any qualitative data into monetary values as well as identifying important intangible benefits. The final meeting reviewed the results and discussed and agreed the final report to be submitted to the organisation.

The AI group utilised the 4-D model of appreciative Inquiry in order to answer the main topic for consideration (Fig. 3.2), which was

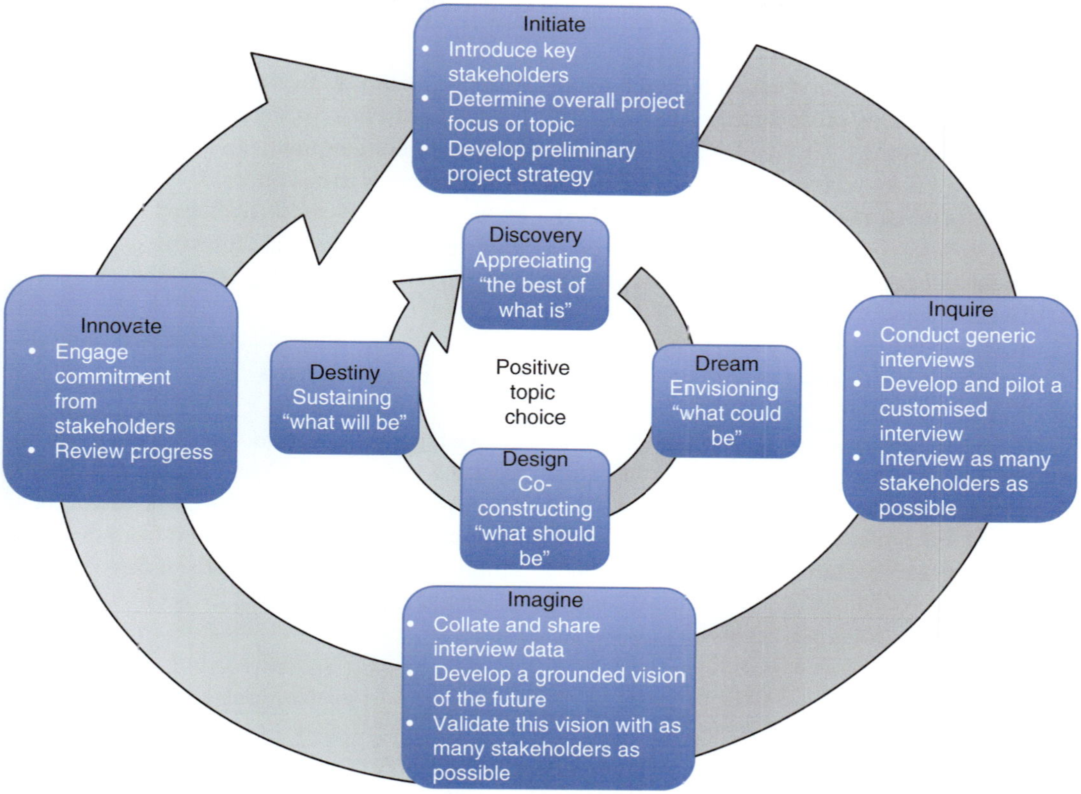

Fig. 3.2 Combined 4D and 4I models (as adapted from Watkins and Mohr [11])

How do we improve the recording of holistic needs assessments and better serve the holistic needs of our patients?

At the initial meeting each member of the AI group was asked to outline their understanding of the reasoning behind the study (the define phase or the affirmative topic), as well as what potential solutions should be considered. In order to explore the 'Discovery' and 'Dream' phases, the group was asked four questions as outlined by Cooperrider, Whitney and Stavros [12]:

1. Think of a high point in your work or experience in the organisation
2. Whilst being modest, what is that you most value about yourself, your work and the organisation?
3. What do you experience as the core factors that give life to this organisation? and without which you think the organisation would cease to exist?
4. Finally, what three wishes would you like to have to heighten the health and vitality of our organisation?

During the initial meeting, metrics for measurement were also discussed and included:

Hard data (as defined by Buzachero et al. [13])

1. Number of holistic needs assessments (SPARC tool) completed
2. Number of follow-up patients seen by the CNS during the pilot study
3. Number of extra 'new' patients seen by Consultant during the pilot study
4. The extra revenue generated through tariff by the Consultant seeing extra 'new' patients

5. The cost of the advanced nurse practitioner course
6. Costs incurred from use of additional resources such as office space and additional secretarial typing

Soft data (as defined by Buzachero et al. [13])

1. Patient satisfaction scores as well as qualitative comments
2. CNS satisfaction/engagement scores as well as qualitative comments

Once the metrics to be collected were defined and agreed upon, an action plan was generated for individual members with data collection methods agreed and how the data would be collected and by whom (Table 3.1).

3.3 Pre-Pilot Questionnaire

Baseline metrics were collected prior to the study to act as a baseline for any change to be compared to. A pre-pilot questionnaire allowed patient satisfaction scores to be collected. The use of qualitative comment boxes also allowed for themes to be generated which would form discussion points at the focus group meeting (Fig. 3.3).

3.4 Focus Group

Themes generated from the comments boxes from the questionnaire were explored further in a focus group setting (Fig. 3.4). The use of focus groups allows for data generated from the interaction of a group of people discussing their

Table 3.1 Data collection plan as agreed by action group members

Level	Pilot objectives	Measure	Data collection method	Data sources	Duration
1	**Reaction**				
	Reaction of patients to the idea of a pilot	Current patient satisfaction scores (8 out of 10)	Questionnaire Focus group	Patients	30 days
2	**Learning**				
	CNS completes advance nurse practice course Group and other healthcare professionals/management must understand reason for pilot	Completion of course with award of certificate (100%)	Certificate of competency	CNS Action group, other healthcare professionals and senior management	6 months 30 days
3	**Application**				
	CNS should start seeing patients independently (following period of mentorship), but with Consultant (CON) support	Checklist	Data monitoring Logbook	Clinic activity records	20 outpatient clinics
4	**Impact**				
	Patients must express value of nurse led clinic at end of pilot Increase in clinic patient number activity	Patient satisfaction scores of at least 8 out of 10 Increase in clinic activity by 20%	Questionnaire Data monitoring	Patients Clinic activity records	30 days 20 outpatient clinics
5	**ROI**				
	Achieve 20% ROI	Comparison to baseline data **plus** non-deterioration of patient satisfaction scores			

Evaluation purpose: Measure impact of pilot
Project: Nurse led clinic pilot
Responsibility: Directorate of General Surgery
Date: 2015/2016

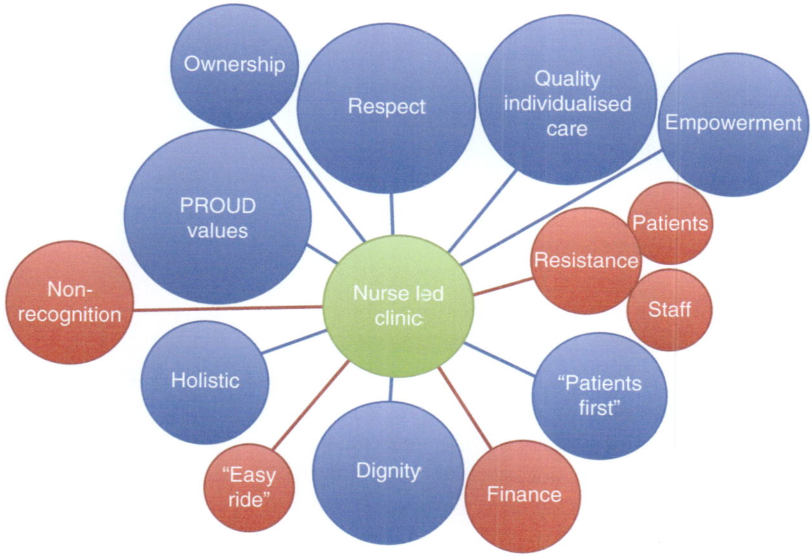

Fig. 3.3 Thematic map representing the themes raised by the AI group, where the size of the balloon represents the relative number of themes coded from the responses

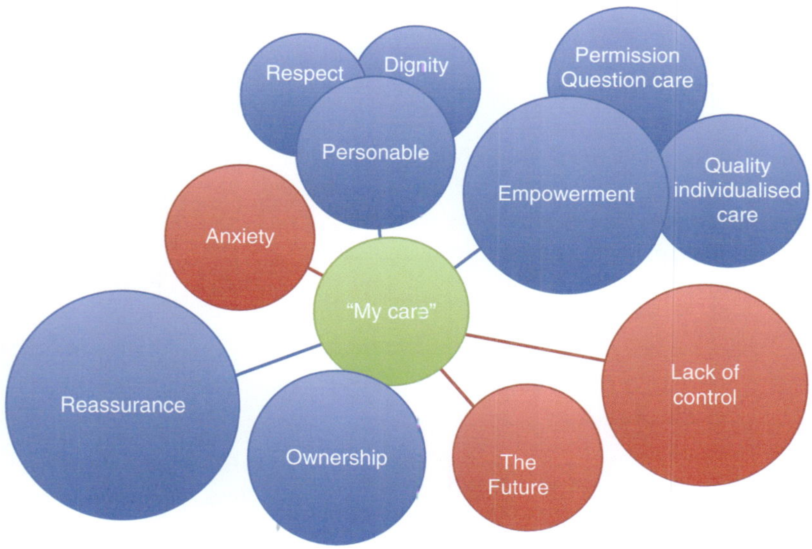

Fig. 3.4 Thematic map representing the themes raised by the focus group, where the size of the balloon represents the relative number of themes coded from the responses

experiences and the themes generated from the questionnaire survey [14].

3.5 Pilot

3.5.1 Inclusion and Exclusion Criteria

Patients were selected sequentially in review date order as long as there was no specific ongoing clinical problems or complications following surgery that required Consultant input. Patients were also excluded from the pilot if they were too frail or wish to be followed up at their local hospital.

3.5.2 Nurse-Led Clinic Pilot Protocol

The pilot follow-up clinic was ran by the CNS using agreed clinical guidelines with a consultant oesophago-gastric surgeon (CON) running a parallel clinic available for advice. This provided a safety-netting mechanism for the CNS during the pilot and also allowed immediate decision-making if required.

3.5.3 Control Group

In order to isolate any confounding factors, a control group was also identified as suggested by Phillips and Phillips [4]. The control group being those patients being seen in the standard Consultant delivered clinics. Hard and soft data metrics were also collected from the control group to be compared with the pilot study intervention group at the end of the study, to determine whether there were any differences between the two groups.

3.5.4 Data Analysis

The AI group and focus group discussions were transcribed verbatim. Coding of the transcripts was undertaken to determine thematic analysis [15] with recurring themes of discussions categorised [16].

3.6 Return on Investment Calculations

Themes generated from the action group are shown in Fig. 3.3 and pre-pilot questionnaire and focus group were triangulated and are shown in Fig. 3.4.

During the focus group, the specific question of nurse-led clinics was also asked, in particular reference to their opinions and concerns with the overwhelming response being positive.

The CNS reviewed 12 patients during the study period.

3.6.1 Current Tariff

Tariff code	WF01B	WF02B	WF01A	WF02A
Description	New patient seen by either doctor **or** CNS	New patient seen by doctor **and** CNS	Follow-up patient seen by either doctor **or** CNS	Follow-up patient seen by doctor **and** CNS
Income	£113	£144	£81	£101

3.6.2 Potential Income from Clinics

	Consultant		CNS	
	WF01B	WF01A	WF01A	Income
Pilot clinic	12 @ £113 £1356	5 @ £81 £405	4 @ $81 £324	**£2085**
Standard clinic	8 @ £113 £904	9 @ £81 £729	0	**£1633**
Potential additional income per pilot clinic				**£452**

3.6.3 Pilot Benefits and Costs

- Quantitative **benefit** metrics:

Item	Benefit
Number of holistic needs assessments completed	**100%** (baseline value pre-pilot was 70%
Total number of new patients seen by Consultant during pilot	**12**
(ai) Income generation by Consultant seeing new patients during pilot	**£1356**
Number of follow-up patients seen by CNS during pilot	**12**
(bi) Income generation by CNS seeing follow-up patients during pilot	**£972**

Item	Benefit
(ci) Potential income generation by both CNS and Consultant seeing follow-up patients as part of MDT assessment during pilot	**£1212**
Total income during pilot study	**ai + bi = £2328** **ai + ci = £2568**

- Quantitative **cost** metrics:

Item	Cost
(a) Cost of initial CNS training (Advance nurse practitioner course)—one-off cost	**£1200**
(b) Annual CNS salary, increment from Band 6 to Band 7	**£5031** to **£6088** (depending on starting point on banding pay scale)
(c) Hourly CNS rate, increment from Band 6 to Band 7	**Band 6 £13.32–£17.84 per hour** **Band 7 £15.89–£20.81 per hour** (Data obtained from RCN website 2016 and confirmed by human resources, STH)
(e) Number of hours utilised by CNS (Band 7) seeing follow-up patients	**30 minutes per patient** 12 patients = 6 hours **£95.34** to **£124.86**
(f) Cost of utilizing clinic room	**£0** (as the cost is automatically deducted from revenue via TIFF (transfer of internal funding formula) which approximates to 49.5% of each patient clinic appointment, to cover the Trust's overhead and maintenance costs
(g) Cost of Band 3 typing support typing up 12 additional letters during pilot	**Band 3 £11.35** to **£13.28 per hour** (Data obtained and revised from NHS Employers website 2016)
(h) Number of hours utilised by typing support (Band 3) typing up CNS follow-up patients	**15 minutes per patient letter** 12 patients = 3 hours **£34.05** to **£39.84**
Total initial set-up and running cost for pilot study	**a + e + f + h = £1329.39** to **£1364.70**

Qualitative Parameters:

Patient satisfaction scores
CNS job satisfaction score

The number of holistic needs assessments completed rose from a benchmark value of 70–100%.

Patient satisfaction scores as assessed against benchmarked pre-pilot questionnaire evaluation showed no deterioration in satisfaction scores, with numerous qualitative comments praising and valuing the CNS nurse-led clinic, which allowed for earlier sign-posting of patients to appropriate services.

"…can't fault it"

"I've never felt rushed"

"Never minded waiting…"

"I wouldn't be concerned to see [CNS] *and if* [she] *was concerned, then I'd be able to see* [the Consultant]"

CNS satisfaction scores improved following establishment of CNS nurse-led clinics.

Another advantage of the CNS nurse-led clinic was to allow the medical team to prioritize seeing those patients that required their specialist input and management, yet allowing routine follow-up patients to spend more quality time with the CNS.

3.6.4 Analysis

Benefit:cost ratio and ROI calculations are based on conservative values of a non-MDT clinics (WF01A and WF01B) tariffs and the higher band CNS and typing support hourly costs.

3.6.5 Benefit: Cost Ratio Calculation

Benefit cost ratio (BCR) = Income/cost.

BCR (using conservative values) = ai + bi/a + e + f = £2328/£1364.70 = **1.71**.

A calculated BCR of 1.71 means that for every £1 spent during the pilot, the income the pilot generated was £1.71.

3.6.6 ROI Calculation

The ROI calculation (using conservative values of lowest income and highest cost) was:

ROI(%) = (Total income − total costs/total costs) × 100

ROI(%) = (£2328 − £1364.70/£1364.70) × 100 = 70.58%

As such the calculated return on investment during the pilot study, where 12 cancer follow up patients were seen and 12 new patients were seen by a Consultant equated to a approximately 71%. Which is the same as the BCR, in that for every £1 spent the net gain (profit) was 71p.

Potentially more important benefits were the intangible benefits, which included:

- An increased completion rate of holistic needs assessments which would satisfy cancer peer review requirements as well as appropriate sign-posting of patients to other services in line with the cancer survivorship initiative.
- Patients continued to be satisfied with the service finding the nurse-led clinic an acceptable alternative to a doctor delivered clinic.
- There was greater job satisfaction for the CNS (which could translate to staff (and knowledge/experience) retention within the Trust.

Another potential impact of a CNS nurse-led clinic, although not formally assessed could be that by signposting patients to appropriate service before a 'crisis' occurs, could potentially save unnecessary admissions to A&E and inpatient beds or extra hospital or GP clinic appointments.

Conclusion

This Quality Improvement project was undertaken with a specific objective to evaluate the ROI through a model of collective and joint working with stakeholders. ROI cannot be calculated as an afterthought and must be part of the overall objectives of the Quality Improvement project. The final calculated value of ROI analysis suggests a net positive gain in income of approximately 71% with benefits of increased completion rates of holistic needs assessments, increased Clinical Nurse Specialist job satisfaction and maintained patient satisfaction rates.

References

1. Phillips JJ, Phillips PP. Return on investment measures success. Ind Manag. 2006;48(2):18–23.
2. Phillips JJ. Handbook of training evaluation and measurement methods. 3rd ed. Boston: Butterworth-Heinemann; 1997.
3. Kirkpatrick DL. Evaluating training programs: the four levels. San Francisco: Berrett-Koehler; 1994.
4. Phillips PP, Phillips JJ. ROI fundamentals: why and when to measure return on investment. San Francisco: Pfeiffer; 2008.
5. National Cancer Survivorship Initiative (NCSI). Assessment and care planning. London: NHS Improvement; 2010.
6. Canter R. Impact of reduced working time on surgical training in the United Kingdom and Ireland. Surgeon. 2011;9(Suppl. 1):S6–7.
7. Samuels M et al. Waiting times for suspected and diagnosed cancer patients: 2015–16 annual report. London: NHS England; 2016.
8. Campbell NC, et al. Secondary prevention in coronary heart disease: a randomised trial of nurse led clinics in primary care. Heart. 1998;80:447–52.
9. Moore S, et al. Nurse led follow up and conventional medical follow up in management of patients with

lung cancer: randomised trial. BMJ. 2002; 325(7377):1145–7.
10. Hoare KJ, Mills J, Francis K. The role of Government policy in supporting nurse-led care in general practice in the United Kingdom, New Zealand and Australia: an adapted realist review. J Adv Nurs. 2012; 68(5):963–80.
11. Watkins J, Mohr B. Appreciative inquiry: change at the speed of imagination. San Francisco: Jossey-Bass; 2001.
12. Cooperrider DL, Whitney D, Stavros JM. Appreciative inquiry handbook: for leaders of change. 2nd ed. Brunswick: Crown Custom Publishing; 2008.
13. Buzachero VV, et al. Measuring ROI in healthcare. New York: McGraw Hill Education; 2013.
14. Kitzinger J. Qualitative research. Introducing focus groups. BMJ. 1995;311(7000):299–302.
15. Saks M, Allsop J. Researching health: qualitative, quantitative and mixed methods. London: Sage; 2007.
16. Saunders M, Lewis P, Thornhill A. Research methods for business students. 4th ed. Pearson Education Ltd: Harlow; 2007.

Effective Medical Leaders Achieving Transformational Change

4

Martin A. Koyle

Healthcare is a dynamic and fast moving ***business***, where never before has leadership been so important to effectively transform healthcare systems. Healthcare costs continue to be driven up with increased demand, an aging population with complex and multiple conditions and advances in technology. Disruptive innovation affects many aspects of healthcare, whether it's new technology such as the robot in surgery, the electronic health record, or the PACS systems, not to mention external influences such as payment systems (government). This results in a changing landscape of priorities, from one based mostly on a production system, to the current concept of one based on value (Value (V) = quality (Q)/cost ($)). Medical school does not prepare its doctors to become leaders. However many individual's demonstrate leadership against these odds. For example, Toby Cosgrove M.D. [1] the world renowned cardiac surgeon turned CEO of the multi-billion dollar enterprise, the Cleveland Clinic, in his preface to his book ***The Cleveland Clinic Way,*** admits "I wasn't born to be a CEO." He reflects that because he grew up as an undiagnosed dyslexic that perhaps that was a blessing in disguise, as he never "fell prey to the herd mentality."

This chapter explores the transformation of healthcare through the development of leadership capability, particularly of its medical leaders, outlining the need for a more deliberate and conscious preparation of doctors to transform healthcare for the future.

Reflecting on my own development through my formative years, while at school, I was probably like most readers, where we strive to 'fit-in' and to be part of the group. In my class I can recall that there was an individual who one might consider the weak one, different with few friends, consistently left out, and often bullied. Ethan was that boy in my class. When I was to have my seventh birthday party, my mother asked why I wanted to invite my entire class to my party with the exception of Ethan. I responded that he didn't fit in. My mother stated that it takes courage to challenge perception and in this case prejudice, and she insisted that I invite him. I lost nothing in the exchange, and perhaps gained respect from other classmates, when it's really Mother who deserved the latter for pushing the point of empathy and inclusion. That was an important landmark for me by realizing my mother wasn't afraid to stand up and be different, and this demonstrated her courage in teaching me a valuable lesson about the ethics of leadership and equality.

M.A. Koyle
Professor of Surgery, School of Medicine and Faculty, IHPME and C-QuIPS, University of Toronto, Toronto, ON, Canada

Women's Auxiliary Chair in Urology and Regenerative Medicine and Chief, Division of Paediatric Urology, The Hospital for Sick Children, Toronto, ON, Canada
e-mail: Martin.Koyle@sickkids.ca

P. Godbole et al. (eds.), *Why Hospitals Fail*, DOI 10.1007/978-3-319-56224-7_4

Simplistically, leadership is about one person's skills in influencing others, while recognizing that the ethical and moral responsibility of such a role is immense. The concept of transformation is based on the importance of the team and unified vision and aims. In healthcare, one must be aware of the system itself, knowing that leaders may range from healthcare assistants to CEO. However even without a title, leadership skills are important, as medicine is not an individual sport, it's a team sport, with considerably more at stake than a sporting match. It is important to distinguish between manager and leader. They may be intertwined in a given role, and can be complimentary. One can be a strong leader and at the same time a poor manager, and vice versa. Kotter [2] has defined management as dealing with complexity whereas leadership is defined as coping with change. Good managers reduce chaos and maximize order. Effective leaders realize change is inevitable and what was commonplace yesterday may be replaced tomorrow. The more volatile the situation, the more that is demanded from leadership.

4.1 Human Nature Is a Reality

> Success is a journey, not a destination. It requires constant effort, vigilance, and evaluation—Mark Twain

The Myers-Briggs Type Indicator (MBTI) is one of the most popular personality tests used by global business and the healthcare sector to assess senior and future leaders. However, there are also many freely available online leadership diagnostic tools (for example, [3]) all of which serve to provide a vehicle for self-awareness and reflection which is seen as the most important element of becoming an effective leader [4]. The MBTI questionnaire has 93 questions, based on the psychologist Carl Jung's work and divides staff into 16 distinct types and combinations of introverts, extroverts, thinkers, feelers, the judging or perceptive. MBTI challenges the myth that extroverts make better leaders than introverts and offers insights into the strengths of different personality types in the workplace. A tool that enables reflection on self seeks to develop an understanding and appreciation of the talents of other work colleagues and supports the more effective delegation of tasks to those employees who will be more happier and satisfied in these particular areas. Self-awareness teaches us that we are not all the same and neither should we be, as we need different personality types within our healthcare teams. Each time I've taken a Myers-Briggs test, I realize that as an ENTP (extrovert, intuition, thinking, perception) I am different from others who also have taken the same test who may be introverted (I), and/or be more sensing (S) and/or prone to feeling (F) and judgment (J). In my limited readings, my personality is associated with leadership potential, but limited management skills. "We" ENTPs don't enjoy demanding of others, because we hate it when it's done to us; fortunately we are allegedly good delegators. We can always learn the skills required to develop as effective leaders but we need the space and time to do this. Once we are aware of our default style and our shortcomings we can steer our own development and support others to do the same.

It's imperative as a good leader to understand what makes us similar and different, and essentially, what drives us! Maslow (1943) (Fig. 4.1) has described our primitive nature with his hierarchy of needs. We all have the basic need of survival, and we all wish to have a true purpose in

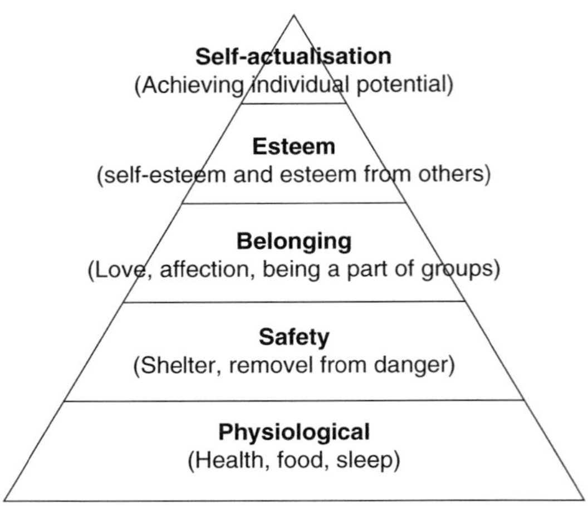

Fig. 4.1 Maslow's hierarchy of needs [5]

life. At the highest level we hope that fulfillment can be attained by achieving our full potential. What makes one individual tick may be totally different from his peer(s). Heifitz and Laurie [6] has proposed the concept of ***adaptive leadership*** knowing that we all have our own comfort zones where we are highly functional. Using the analogy of a pot on a stove, some may need the heat turned up while others require that it be turned down in order to reach the sweet spot of optimal function.

As a doctor, we are inherently placed in leadership roles, and have a responsibility to understand and form positive relationships with individual team members who represent our stakeholder networks. Of course a lot depends upon one's leadership position and the type of relationship one has with an individual will impact on the level and type of influence possible, within the too often present hierarchy of that institution. So for instance in my "official" position, I am directly responsible for the surgeons and trainees, as well as those under our payroll, in my small division. This represents a hybrid of management and leadership. However, I am indirectly in a position of ***leadership*** for those outside my direct realm, the individuals in the operating room or clinic environment and even physicians of other disciplines. The latter is a unique potential leadership responsibility for all doctors, even without title, and the key is in the word team. If we have a common aim of delivering 'value based care', and this message is only transmitted vertically from the top down in the "siloed" environment of a hospital, it makes it much more difficult to lead effectively in the organization to deliver quality patient care to all. Patients move across the organization vertically and a good leader needs to work to support vertical and horizontal communication and team working to support a quality patient experience.

Regardless of our environment, within a medical system we thus focus our aim on our primary customer, the patient. Having that common focus, assists us in innovating and developing new strategies as a response to patient and other constituent stakeholder feedback. It allows opportunities to create standard work and "work smarter, not harder". With value being a central theme of modern healthcare, processes can not only be instituted, they can be managed more efficiently, and most importantly, be measured. Remember that if Value is Q/$, then establishing metrics to measure patient focused improvement is paramount if we are to attain a culture of continuous improvement and not be managed by financial targets. We must hold ourselves accountable to delivering quality services to patients providing value for money to all our stakeholders.

Many of the concepts of ***Lean***, that have been translated from industry to healthcare such as best practices, standardization and eliminating waste with the aim of improving productivity and efficiency, are not necessarily novel and were recognized well over a century ago by Frederick Taylor [7]. Within healthcare and with the drive to develop effective teamworking, we are also aware of the nuances of context for staff. Some environments are particularly stressful and having some variability in the process in terms of breaks for staff and flexible rotas are ways of building in support, kindness and valuing the workforce. It is important to support staff to have breaks during the working day in order to reduce fatigue, stress and maintain emotional fitness. Fortes-Mayer [8] argues that emotional fitness is as important as physical fitness and is the speed with which you return to peace and love once you have been upset, scared or angry. It is argued that employees need support to think deeply about themselves and how they respond to situations in the workplace and that this helps to realise potential. We now know that breaks are necessary for the benefit of workers, to maintain morale and to produce energy and creativity to improve the quality of services to patients.

Medicine in and of itself is inherently stressful. Increasingly, such stresses are compounded by escalating worry related to complaints and potentially even to litigation, that are perceived to be a result of our performance or actions. Historically, the healthcare environment has been a culture of blame. Lucian Leape [9] aptly stated that: "The single greatest impediment to error prevention in the medical industry is that we punish people for making mistakes." The Institute of Medicine [10] released the important publication of ***To Err is Human.*** Although this is preached across the world, for many healthcare professionals, the belief is that blame and scapegoating remain omnipresent. Actions can speak louder than words. Systems are devised in order to recognize human reality and error. The Swiss Cheese Model [11] promotes that systems must be created that minimize or ideally, eliminate, the potential for all holes in multiple pieces of Swiss cheese to line up perfectly so that an error can pass perfectly through all the holes without being blocked. Burnout is an ever increasing reality in healthcare and leaders must make efforts to minimize this occurrence. It has been stated that 87% of issues that develop between individuals were due to inter-personal communication skills, not those of competence! Being direct and transparent become key attributes of successful leaders [12].

W. Edwards Deming, who revolutionized the Japanese automobile industry after the Second World War, conceived the System of Profound Knowledge. Conceptually this is a Venn diagram incorporating elements: knowledge of a system (understanding the entire process) knowledge of variation (ranges and causes of variation in quality and metrics to analyze them), knowledge of psychology (understanding human nature) and epistemology or the theory of knowledge (concepts that explain what we know and what are limits might be) [13]. The relevance is its applicability to not just the automobile industry but to expand it to others including healthcare in an effort to improve it.

In our definition of Management vs. Leadership, it was emphasized that Kotter [2] felt the latter is pertinent to issues that surround change. In the healthcare environment, change is inevitable and is often resisted. It is commonplace to hear colleagues complain about the new electronic record, or actually avoid learning new techniques. With the advent of laparoscopic cholecystectomy, there were initially few who embraced the technique, but eventually most surgeons realized that the technique was not futuristic, but rather a " disruptive reality" in the rapidly progressive environment of modern healthcare. The challenge for all of us is to work out how such advances can be available to all populations in the developing and developed world and not just accessible to the few.

Finally there were those remaining who continued to ignore this and eventually had to jump on board the proverbial steamroller before they became part of the road. The concept of ***Diffusion of Innovations*** was that of Rogers [14]. In understanding human nature, he felt it was divided into five elements (Fig. 4.2). Innovators are a sparse few (2.5%) while those that seem to jump on board virtually any new

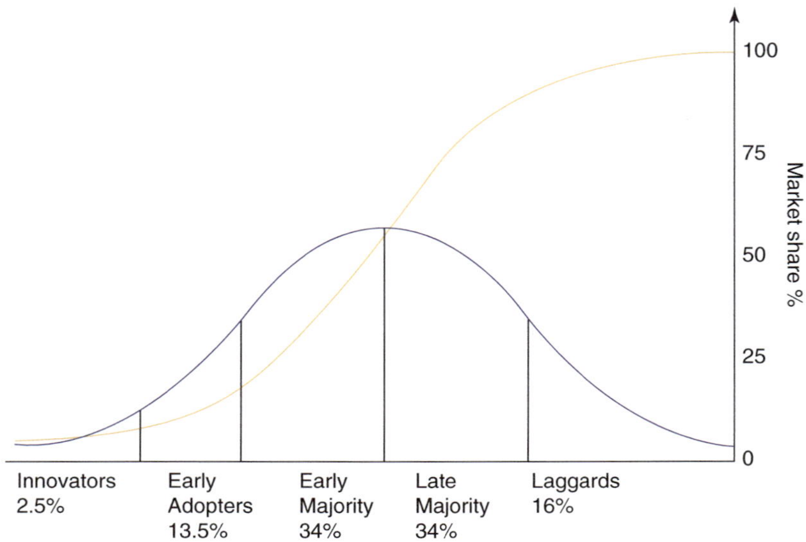

Fig. 4.2 Roger's diffusion of innovations (from the book 'Diffusion of Innovation' first published, by E M Rogers, 1962)

advance without any prodding are the early adopters (13.5%). In order to really promote a change one must engage the early majority (34%) and rapidly as the figure shows an equal number of the late majority (34%), with the remaining 16% being the laggards. This reiterates the importance of galvanizing support from the right stakeholders, at the right time and being cognizant of the System of Profound Knowledge in order to promote change. Kotter [15] has summarized eight pivotal points that are important in leading change:

1. Creating urgency
2. Creating the guiding coalition
3. Developing a vision
4. Communicating that vision
5. Empowering others to act on that vision
6. Generating short-term wins
7. Consolidating gains & producing more change
8. Anchoring (institutionalizing) new approaches in the culture

In addition, he suggests that there are strategic choices that leaders must consider when promoting change:

1. How directive or participative to be, i.e. *how much* to involve others?
2. *Who* will you involve???
3. How fast to go?
4. How much time to give yourself?

Reflecting on the points above, it is imperative for a leader to have an aim and communicate this to all stakeholders, but also to achieve long term gain by acknowledging success and rewarding those involved. This becomes most important in sustaining and growing these gains. Ideally the leader recognizes the importance of using "we" rather than "I" when promoting change. Humility can go a long way. There is no set time as to how long a project should take. It is important to be efficient and follow timelines and deadlines and that these are visible and open to team members. This allows progress to be monitored by all involved.

4.2 Why Aren't We Always Successful in Implementing Change?

Leadership is an entity that requires work and knowledge. Despite one's best efforts however, even good leaders fail in impacting change. This can be frustrating and demoralizing, requiring reflection on the importance of inter-communication.

Three decades ago, Ambrose [16] described five components that are interactive in promoting change: visions, skills, incentives, resources and an action plan. In healthcare, the game plan in a hierarchal system is ever changing. Likewise, fiscal support becomes a major issue, especially if a project is large and takes time. We all know about the revolving door of administrators and hence philosophies at our institutions. This can be tumultuous and affect even the most researched action plan. Incentives are visibly lacking and many team members ask what is in it for them? Altruism only goes so far. Perhaps the most important component is vision, which must be clear and logical and well communicated.

Golden [17] has identified four stages of transforming healthcare organizations. First one must determine the desired end state (vision). Secondly, assess the readiness for change. This is a pivotal element that looks at the system past and present, engages not only the stakeholders and patients but the reality of executive and senior administrative support. Communicating and reinforcing the benefits of a proposed change can broaden support. Simultaneously as part of the third step, goals and tasks can be revisited and organizational re-design can ensue. The last step is reinforcing and sustaining change, which will include showcasing and fine tuning the project with recognition and reward of team members.

4.3 Illustrative Example

Never argue with a fool.
Onlookers may not be able to tell the difference—
Mark Twain

At my current institution I was amazed that 14 different surgeons from two services performed pediatric hernia repairs. The same operation, which rarely takes more than 30–45 min, had anywhere between 51 and 96 instruments on a tray. Some of the instruments went by different names depending on the surgeon. In each case, although the surgeon may have been constant, trainees and operating theater nurses were not. Different nomenclature and individual surgeon demands could create havoc and opened up opportunities for miscommunication, and potentially for errors.

We aimed to reduce the number of instruments utilized for pediatric hernia repair and standardize instruments to a minimum and to be contained on a single tray for all surgeons. We had to undertake research and do a root cause analysis to identify why the current problem prevailed. Primarily it was a culture of "we always do it this (my) way!"

Importantly we had to identify our stakeholders. Patients are involved in as much as they, or on their referring physician's recommendation, choose to attend our healthcare facility. While this project didn't involve patients directly, we continued to survey patient satisfaction to ensure that the service continued to be one of value and to give us feedback to constantly improve. Knowing what patients value and don't value can steer healthcare transformation. Primary stakeholders for this project included nurses and the staff in central sterilization, who we hoped to engage immediately and hence would become "our early adopters". The surgeons, who we hyposthesized would be late adopters and even laggards (most resistant to change), likely would be easier to persuade to change if these other key stakeholders had already embraced the change. We first surveyed all stakeholders for an initial appraisal of their feelings and perceptions regarding the project's aim. We also encouraged open communication at any time with me in the role as project lead. Throughout the project each stakeholder group was revisited repeatedly to update status and provide answers to any queries they may have had.

We trained four observers who watched each of the 14 surgeons perform a minimum of two cases each and count the instruments that were actually used in each operation. By doing so, we were able to construct a single standardized tray composed of only 28 instruments that had been used in >50% of all cases observed. Hence even the smallest tray was reduced by almost 50%. A follow up survey demonstrated uniform satisfaction by all stakeholders and >90% felt the process was sustainable and should be rolled out to other common surgeries. In addition, the final tray was >50% less weight than the largest trays used previously providing a potential ergonomic benefit and the cycle time to count, process and sterilize and re-package each tray was reduced significantly, creating a fiscal benefit.

In summary, leadership in healthcare is a path that is serpentine because of continuous change and a need of for continuous improvement and transformation. We know that the more effective leaders are those who develop and refine more self-awareness [4] and understand their personality and representative default style while recognizing the multiple differences of the potential stakeholders. This allows an effective leader to use a range of styles, and constantly reflect upon their effectiveness to engage and influence others. There is a need to constantly develop through opportunities presented in the workplace, continuously to gain new skills and experience. It is a challenging era for physicians as leaders as the internet allows patients to become 'experts' of their own condition and knowledgeable with respect to various medical conditions, disruptive technology impacts not only clinical practice but how we interact in medicine communication, and external forces continue to analyze our value within the system. It is imperative that future leaders are cognizant of the importance of quality and have the tools available including identifying appropriate metrics that support evaluation of cost, and ways to measure the value to patients in terms of patient safety and the quality of experience.

References

1. Cosgrove T. The Cleveland Clinic Way: lessons in excellence from one of the World's Leading Healthcare Organizations. New York: McGraw-Hill; 2014.
2. Kotter JP. What leaders really do. HBR. 2001;25–34.
3. Northouse PG. Leadership theory and practice. Thousand Oaks: Sage Publications; 2007.
4. Goleman D. Leadership that gets results. Harv Bus Rev. 2000;78(2):78–90.
5. Maslow AH. A theory of human motivation. Psychol Rev. 2014;50(4):370–96.
6. Heifitz RA, Laurie DL. The work of leadership. Harv Bus Rev. 2001;79(11):37–47.
7. Kanigel R. The one best way: Frederick Winslow Taylor and the enigma of efficiency. New York: Penguin-Viking; 1997.
8. Fortes-Mayer T. The freemind experience: the three pillars of absolute happiness. London: Watkins Publishing Ltd; 2015.
9. Leape LL Errors in medicine. Clin Chim Acta. 2009;404(1):2–5.
10. Kohn LT, Corrigan JM, Donaldson MS. To err is human building a safer health system. Washington: Institute of Medicine National Academy Press; 1999.
11. Reason J. The contribution of latent human failures to the breakdown of complex systems. Philos Trans R Soc Lond B Biol Sci. 1990;327:475–84.
12. Kachalia A. Improving patient safety through transparency. N Engl J Med. 2013;369:1677–9.
13. Deming WE. Out of the crisis. Cambridge: MIT Press; 2000.
14. Rogers EM. Diffusion of innovations. 5th ed. New York: Simon and Schuster; 2003.
15. Kotter JP. Leading change. Cambridge: HBR Press; 2010.
16. Ambrose D. Managing complex change. Pittsburgh: The Enterprise Group, Ltd; 1987.
17. Golden B Transforming healthcare organizations. Healthc Q. 2006;10(sp):10–9.

A Critique of Conceptual Leadership Styles'

5

Bolarinde Ola

5.1 Introduction

In this chapter, I aim to review the literature and published research on the old and new concepts of leadership, emotional intelligence; and the impacts on group and individual performances. I will specifically critique the literature with an understanding of its relevance to 'Why Hospitals Fail'. One of the major difficulties with the current volume of leadership theory is that it is often explored as a concept devoid of context, of history, organizational culture and with very little emphasis on the quality of health care. Indeed there is often reference to a lack of leadership in inquiry reports, but what is meant by this concept is often ambiguous and lacking of a consistently understood definition.

5.2 Leadership

Over the past 40 years or so, there have been many opinions about leadership, as a result of which there are hundreds of definitions [1, 2]. Over time, the common theme is that leaders can transform their concepts, convictions and vision into organisational changes through their influence over other people ([3, 4], p. 286). The story of the world has, very frequently, been synonymous with the story of its leaders, whether good or bad. For example, the biblical story of the exodus is incomplete without the historical accounts of Rameses, Moses and Joshua; and neither can accounts of the Second World War ever be separated from the histories of Hitler, Churchill, Stalin or Roosevelt. Each is a study in leadership theory, leadership styles, emotional intelligence, achievements and failures as reflected directly or otherwise in various styles described by Goleman [5] as democratic authoritative, pace-setting, affiliative, coaching and coercive (A summary of leadership theor y is presented in Fig. 5.1). However more recent contributions of leadership have critiqued the ambiguity of the concept and called for more application to the context of practice with more calls for explaining 'leadership work' (Blom and Alvesson, 2015). It is the inter-relationship between style, approach and context that can be most useful when considering the major issues and challenges for hospitals which are: to move towards a more integrated model of health care delivery, more focus on prevention, safer surgery check-lists, minimally invasive surgical interventions, enhanced recovery programmes, enhanced multi disciplinary inputs to services, access to self directed approaches to health care, and self/group empowerment approaches.

B. Ola
Sheffield Teaching Hospitals NHS Foundation Trust, University of Sheffield, Sheffield, UK
e-mail: Bola.Ola@sth.nhs.uk

P. Godbole et al. (eds.), *Why Hospitals Fail*, DOI 10.1007/978-3-319-56224-7_5

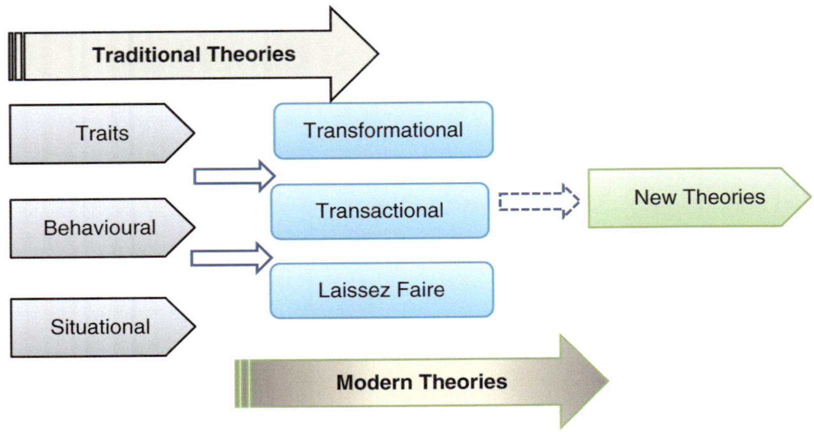

Fig. 5.1 The development of leadership theories

5.3 Traditional Theories of Leadership

Traditionally it was, for many years, considered that some people were born to lead because they inherited traits and qualities found in leaders [6]. Early research, therefore, focused on three theories: Trait, behavioural and contingency/situational approaches to leadership.

5.3.1 Traits and Leadership

Early research concluded that many leaders had personality and psychological traits, which were inherited, but transferrable from one situation to another [7–11]. Such desirable traits included an extrovert personality, charisma; masculinity and dominance. Other researchers like Senior and Fleming [12] have however identified emotional intelligence and conservatism as preferable traits. Traditional theories suffer from criticisms that they are difficult to test robustly and have narrow generalisability. For example trait theory focuses too much on physical and personality characteristics like domineering masculinity, charisma, extrovertness and conservatism [13, 14]. Apart from a disagreement on the important traits, it also suffers from the weakness of not being tested against influences of gender equality, socio-cultural and geopolitical differences across regions; or against confounding effects of job training and professional development [14, 15].

5.3.2 Behavioural Leadership

As the validity of the trait theory became increasingly questioned, there was a move towards an investigation of how behaviours, not personal traits, influenced whether leaders succeeded or failed [16, 17]. Such behavioural research led to several leadership models including the McGregor's Theory [18], the Ohio State University of Michigan Models [19], and the Managerial Grid Model of Blake and Mouton [20]. Behavioural theorists can be criticised for focusing on laboratory and field data, which not only detached from workplace reality, thereby limiting generalisability; but also for an inability to explain how effective behaviours in one situation translated to unsuccessful outcomes in other circumstances.

5.3.3 Situational Approach

In time, further research sought to improve understanding of leadership styles in the face of evolving challenges. Several theories were formed to explain how effective leaders change their styles according to situations and contingencies, as they arise. These theories, including Fielder's contingency theory of leadership, the path-goal theory of leader effectiveness, Hersey and Blanchard's life-cycle theory, the cognitive resource theory, and the decision process theory [2, 8, 21, 22] which were based on studies of leaders under different situations. They concluded that good leaders can respond to situations around them and that leadership performance can also be enhanced or diminished by resources available. It can therefore be argued that a woman with excellent leadership skills should succeed, whether heading the Global Health Unit of the Royal College of Obstetricians and Gynaecologists in London or a World Health Organisation unit in Nigeria, West Africa. On the contrary, another person may lead effectively in London and not able to respond to socio-cultural barriers against women leaders in other countries. The Mid Staffordshire Hospital inquiry (Francis 2013) reveals what happens when a hospital forgets it is in the business of providing quality health care. Secondments of general managers and managers from the non-health sectors like M&S-a leading retail chain in the UK, may not necessarily contribute to the success of a hospital in difficulty; and in many ways the difficulties of the NHS may be further compounded by a lack of clinical balance at the executive board—where non-clinical personnel dominate particularly in the NHS.

5.4 Modern Perspectives of Leadership

Modern organizations have changed significantly in size and complexity over time and so also have the skills and styles of leadership required for the modern day organisation. Over time, it has become difficult to apply traditional leadership theories to the functions and survival of huge national and multinational organizations, including the healthcare sector. More recently, research has focused on two main modern theories of leaderships: transformational and transactional [19, 23–27]. This general compartmentalization of leadership styles into two or three have however been criticized. Blom and Alvesson [28] describe "hegemonic ambiguity" of leadership definitions; and particularly the didactic, within-leadership concepts which narrows everything into convenient transformational, transactional or Laissez-faire styles [19, 23]. There is also significant pan-disciplinary vagueness which tends to portray each of these styles as one-size-fit-all professional situations. To illustrate, Hu et al. [29] found that a transformational approach was most effective leadership style of surgeons in an operating theatre (OR). This has however been critiqued on the grounds that modern WHO safer-surgery check-lists, actually requires safe and efficient surgeons to adopt a task-based transactional approach in the OR [30]. Contrary to Hu et al. [29], Parker et al. [31] had found a predominantly task-focused leadership style among theatre staff. Furthermore, not enough has been written about how cultural, religious, and geo-political factors influence the interactions between these broad leadership styles and followership. These issues are very relevant in organizations like the National Health Service, where leadership styles must be constantly adaptable to accommodate ethnic, socio-cultural and geo-political diversities; and religious tolerance.

Another critique of the bland compartmentalization of leadership into two or three widely accepted styles is that new paradigms were largely neglected from close scrutiny. One example is the neo-emergent leadership, which originated from the Oxford school of leadership [32, 33]. Neo-emergent theory describes the use of intelligent information management to account for stewardship to benefit the leader. The practice is widespread, where for example, a leader or other stakeholders use sponsored advertisements, press releases and blogs on social media to create a good impression of leadership. Neo-emergent leadership is also widely practiced within the National Health Service Hospitals, where regular newsletters are circulated to patients, relatives and staff on how the chief executive has led the trust through ground breaking new treatments, services, innovations or research. Surprisingly however, the objective effects of such leadership style on followership performance do not appear to have been researched [30, 34].

Nevertheless, and irrespective of classification, leadership styles do appear to have significant impacts on team processes in the workplace [24, 26, 27]. The Full Range Leadership Development

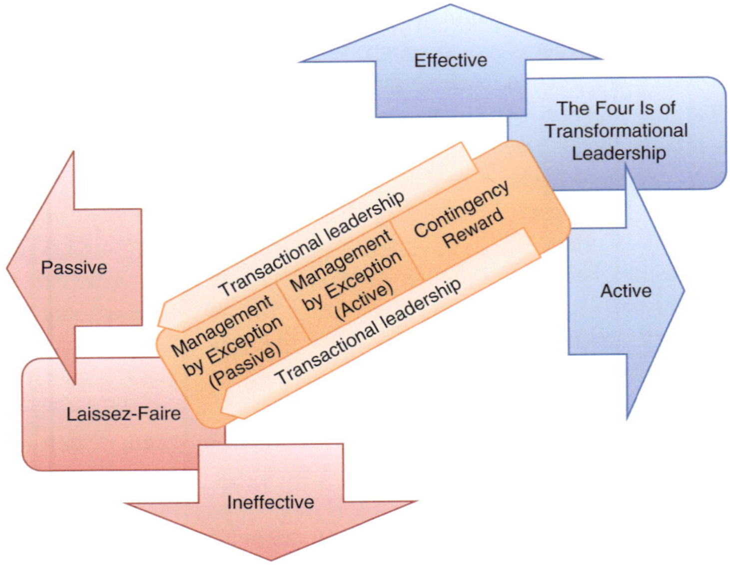

Fig. 5.2 Schematic representation of full range leadership development theory (adapted from [81])

Model by Bass and Avolio (1997) grouped eight leadership criteria into active, passive, effective and ineffective leadership tendencies. These eight criteria are Idealised attributes (IA), Idealised behaviors (IB), inspirational motivation (IM), intellectual stimulation (IS) individual consideration (IC), contingency reward (LR), management by active expectation (MEA) and management by passive expectation (MEP). These four were then regrouped under transformational, transactional or laissez-faire leadership styles [35] (Fig. 5.2).

5.4.1 Transformational Leadership

The Full Range Leadership Development Model identified four criteria characterising the active, effective tendencies of transformational leadership. These are Idealised influence, inspirational motivation, individualised consideration, and intellectual stimulation [35]. Leaders with Charisma (Idealised influences) are role models for their followership. Such leaders are trusted, admired and identified with [35, 36]. Inspirational leaders motivate and inspire members by communicating aims and objectives, and high expectations in simplified, meaningful, but challenging ways [37]. This behaviour can also enrich team spirit and initiative with optimism and zeal [35, 36]. Individualised consideration includes strong tendencies to mentor, support, encourage and coaching followers thereby directing skill acquisition towards future organisational needs and continuing professional development [35, 36, 38, 39]. Transformational leaders also encourage innovation and creativity by stimulating followership to question irrational assumptions, re-define problems and re-approach old challenges in new ways [35].

5.4.2 Transactional Leadership

Transactional leadership is hinged on a carrot and stick principle of benefits for task accomplishments and punishment for poor performance [40], in [23, 41, 42]. Bass and Avolio [35] described transactional leadership as hinging on bureaucratic authority and legitimacy and focused on compliance and task completion.

From the Full Range Leadership Development Model, actions denoting transactional leadership include contingent reward and management by exception. In contingent reward, the leader uses the carrot approach of promises, commendation, and material reward as motivational incentives to push followers towards attaining contractual work performance. In active management-by-exception, the leader directly supervises and intervenes when the follower is deviating away from agreed guidelines or target. By contrast, in passive management-by-exception the leader monitors indirectly and can only intervene when standards are not met [35, 39, 43].

Both styles of leaderships are frequently complementary. Indeed, transactional leadership is entrenched in the curricula of postgraduate medical and surgical training, where trainees are expected to show learning curves in skill acquisition from direct to indirect supervision leading to independent practice. In such a system, transactional leadership offers corrective management either actively on the spot, or passively at quarterly formative assessment meetings. In modern day NHS however, leaders also have to be more emotionally intelligent as they are expected to provide moral leadership, helping and listening skills that form the foundation stones for implementing trust strategic directions; and commitment and dedication by followership [44, 45].

5.5 Emotional Intelligence

There is a vast and confusing number of definitions for emotional intelligence; also called emotional literacy by others [46]. Martinez ([47], p. 72) defines emotional intelligence as "a set of non-cognitive skills, capabilities and competencies that influence a person's ability to cope with environmental demands and pressures". Goleman [48] describes emotional intelligence as the foremost leadership skill, which harnesses four domains: self-awareness, self-management, social awareness and relationship management. Good leaders are aware of self and their physical and social environment, which facilitates how they influence people around them in a positive way. Demonstration of positive emotions like happiness, laughter and optimism can lift workers to achievements and progress; whereas negative emotions like anger, hostility, fear and anxiety can be demoralising to a workforce.

5.6 Theories of Emotional Intelligence

Thorndike [49] is widely credited with the first modern theory of emotional intelligence. He described three types of intelligence: abstract, concrete and social. Abstract intelligence, measured by intelligent quotient measured how clever a person is. Concrete intelligence, he felt was needed for manipulating objects and shapes, and social intelligence that was needed to interact and associate with people evolved into emotional intelligence as we know it today. Other researchers like Howard Gardner [50] and Gardner and Hatch [51], extended the concepts of Thorndike to include other forms of intelligence that were not measurable by intelligent quotient.

The term emotional intelligence was first credited to two psychologists, Peter Salovey and John Mayer [52]. These researchers felt that intellect was separate from emotions and went on to develop a norm-tested emotional quotient tool to complement a pre-existing intelligent quotient test. Peter Salovey and John Mayer [52] suggested that emotional intelligence related to four domains: perceiving, appraising, understanding and managing emotions. The work of Salovey and Mayer led to the development of the ability model and subsequently the Multifactor Emotional Intelligence Scale (MEIS) [53, 54]. The MEIS also called the Mayer-Salovey-Caruso Emotional Intelligence Test (MSCEIT), describes 12 tasks designed to measure a person's ability to perceive, assimilate, understand, and manage emotions [53]. Goleman [5] built on existing work by proposing five components of emotional intelligence; self-awareness, self-management, (self-regulation, self-motivation), social awareness, and social skills, that can have a significant impact on an individual's perception and response to organisational environments. Self-awareness is all about understanding one's likes and dislikes; and one's innate abilities and weaknesses. Self-regulation is the capacity to exercise proportionate control in the face of external influences. Self-motivation describes the ability to keep focused in the pursuit of goals by optimism, resoluteness and commitment. Social awareness is the emotion of empathy or feeling what others feel; an important attribute of a leader in the workplace. Social skills, according to Goleman [5] include effective communication, conflict resolution, collaboration, cooperation, managing change and team building. As a result of his work, a comprehensive 137-item emotional Quotient test was developed to measure the five dimensions described above [5].

More recently, other tools have been developed. Bar-On [55, 56] developed a self-reporting 133-item questionnaire with a five-point rating scale called the Emotional Intelligence Inventory, to generate scores for five emotions: intrapersonal, interpersonal, adaptability, stress management and mood. One of the better-validated tools, the multi-rater Emotional Competency Profiler (ECP) was designed by Wolmarans [57] to measure emotional intelligence using self- and group assessments [58, 59]. Wolmarans [57] multi-rater assessment tool provides feedback that can be beneficial by facilitating self-reflection, and a measure of individual emotions as viewed by other people, thereby highlighting areas of weaknesses and strengths. Seven competencies are measured in Wolmarans ECP. These are self-motivation; self-esteem or self-regard, self-management, change resilience, interpersonal relations integration of 'head and heart' and emotional literacy [46].

5.7 Importance of Emotional Intelligence

Emotional intelligence is an important indicator of a leader's ability to succeed. Many studies link emotional intelligence with individual and group performances in the workplace. Research by Schutte et al. [60] and Huy [61] demonstrated a positive link between emotional intelligence and effective outcomes like optimism, task mastery, mental wellbeing and job satisfaction; but negatively related to symptoms of depression. The impact of emotional intelligence on group performance has also been investigated [62, 63]; with evidence suggesting that emotional intelligence can determine high and average performance in the workplace

So, hospitals fail not because there is a dearth of leadership qualities or competences (emotional literacy, self-esteem, self-management, self-motivation, change resilience, interpersonal relations and integration of head and heart) that define emotionally intelligent leadership. On the contrary, failure arises, because the focus of emotionally competent managers have shifted from safe, qualitative, holistic healthcare to surrogate markers of healthcare like targets, waiting lists, theatre usage. The clinician is highly trained, and wants to provide "platinum quality" healthcare to all his/her patients every time, whereas managers generally push for "silver or bronze quality" healthcare to as many people as possible; and in as little time as feasible. To illustrate lets consider the effect of theatre utilisation tables which is commonly used as measure of NHS operating theatre performance [64]; but highly favoured by managers in some NHS Trusts as surrogate marker of a surgeon's performance. The table summarises the percentage of time a surgeon actually operates out of actual theatre time available. Managers will usually not include the reasons for low utilisation-like patient cancellation at short notice, equipment failures, unavoidable delayed start in theatre, complex surgery or unexpected developments during surgery. A senior surgeon preparing for a job-plan meeting with his clinical director will present patient outcomes like cure rates, complication rates and returns to theatre to justify requests for changes in job plan. At the job-plan meeting, he may be surprised by a different list prepared ahead by managers which focuses instead on his clinic and theatre waiting times and his theatre utilisation rates. So, a request for more resources and operating time by a safe surgeon with excellent feedback, may be denied by managers because his theatre utilisation is low.

5.8 Performance

It is important to discuss performance because the survival, effectiveness and economic performance of any organisation depend on its performance and how this is managed. Organisations are increasingly complex and the measures of performance are therefore multifaceted, ranging from internal factors like assets, human resources and skill-mix goal and target achievements, financial health, profitability, shareholders' returns; to external factors like political environment, taxation, legislation, and other socio-economic factors. In the prevailing environments of stiff competition, it is recognised that some hospitals will close in the next few years as community based models emerge, leaders and Managers are under increasing pressure to improve hospital organisational performance, and this has led to various tools for assessing group performances and individual job appraisals.

5.8.1 Individual Performance in Organisations

Individual performance depends on training qualifications, innate ability, work experience, remuneration, motivation and leadership. Individual performance needs nurturing, irrespective of whether for-profit companies or voluntary non-profit organisations to achieve strategic objectives. Although most employees' tend to aspire to perform to the best of their ability, the desire also has to be nurtured and guided [65]. Managing individual performance has become so important that continuing professional development schemes and yearly assessments and appraisals have become quite commonplace. In the NHS the hospitals are quality assessed in relation to how well their staff are managed as part of the CQC assessment.

5.8.2 Group Performance in Voluntary Non-profit Organisations

The author works with the Nigerian Liaison Group of the Royal College of Obstetricians and Gynaecologist, which is a non-profit, charitable organisation which interacts very closely with the National Health Service. This group, like seven other groups from Bangladesh, Egypt, Ghana, India, Iraq, Pakistan and Sudan, is a collection of people who share the common characteristics of defined membership, group awareness, common purpose, interaction, co-existence and ability to pull in the same direction [2]. Not-for-profit groups usually measure their performance by how well they achieved their operational targets and set goals. Not-for-profit organisations may not have the additional drivers of profitability and shareholder demands to motivate performance. Nevertheless, they have other financial drivers like incomes from donations and grants, expenses and operational costs. To remedy t his Kaplan and Norton [66] and Kaplan [67] introduced the Balanced Scorecard, a performance management system that incorporates financial measurements of progress, complemented by three other measures: value for customers, how well the internal process is running and organisational learning and growth (Fig. 5.3).

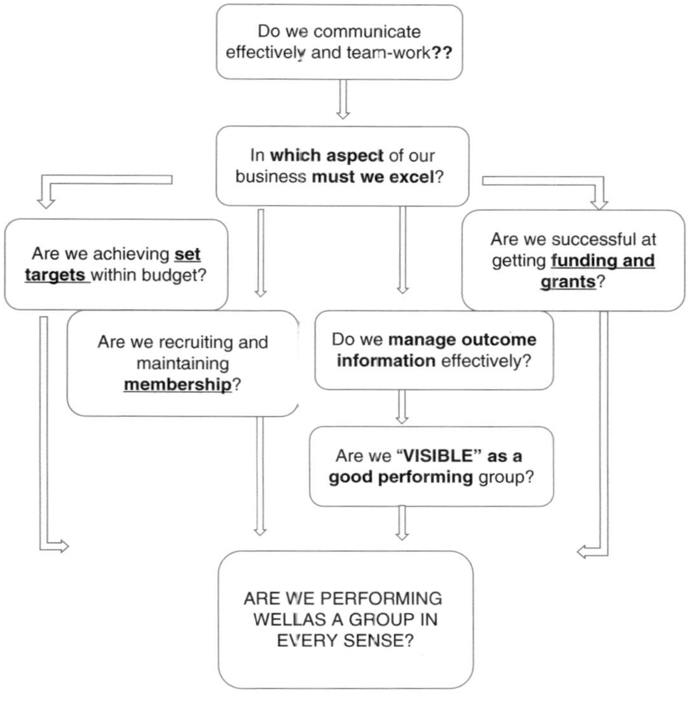

Fig. 5.3 Adapting the balanced scorecard framework to a non-profit group [67]

5.9 Leadership and Performance

There is a consensus that the most important factor in organisational performance is leadership. There is however no doubt that the skills, qualification, motivation, stimulation and dedication of members are also crucial to organisational performance, particularly in voluntary organisations; nevertheless, it is the leader who must be able to harness and optimise these attributes towards a collective goal. An effective leader can enhance the output of the entire workforce by bringing out the best in individuals and collectively [2, 37]. Bass and Avolio [68] demonstrated that transformational leadership has a greater influence on organisational performance when compared with transactional leadership. Other researchers [69] have also concluded that transactional is an extension of transformational leadership; whereas the former brings out the expected performance from a group, the latter can motivate group and individual performance beyond expectations [37, 68]. Furthermore, it is argued that transactional leadership was more suited to organisations engaged in stable markets without rivals or competitions, whereas transformational leaders were more adapted to the modern dynamic marketplace with fierce rivalry and competitions for scarce resources; and more demanding clientele [70].

5.10 Leadership Competencies and Performance in Non-profit Groups

There is relatively little research on leadership styles of medical leaders in workplaces [71–73]; and even less so in non-profit voluntary medical associations [74]. In modern voluntary, not-for-profit organisations the "market", contrary to expectation, can be quite dynamic, with constantly changing and competitive playing field. Although not driven by profit and loss and shareholders, it is influenced by fierce competition for scarce funding, aggressive competitive advertising, and increasingly stringent grants criteria. Therefore, modern voluntary organisations are better off with transformational leaders, who must have vision, be committed and focused on the organisational goals [75]. He or she must also be courageous and willing to challenge the status quo if necessary, and abide by set values that are important to the organisation and the vulnerable public being served [75]. Like counterparts in industry, leaders of voluntary organisations should be professionally competent in areas relevant to the running of their organisation, with, for example, a good understanding of scenario planning and simplified break-even analyses.

5.11 Who Should Be Hospital Leaders?

More doctors need to be supported to move into leadership and management positions in hospitals. The English NHS top executive jobs are managed by non-clinical professionals. There is a need for clinical leadership with more diversity in the top teams to enable effective hospital success. Development in both leadership and management is needed for all doctors and it is now recognised that it is not 'an optional extra' ([76], p. 442). Leadership development must not focus purely on technical competencies, but on the ability to create climates in which individuals can themselves act to improve services and care. Staff at all levels need to be given the skills to have the courage to challenge poor practice and to lead effectively. For the past two decades, attending a recognised leadership and management course was obligatory requirement to completion of specialist training in Obstetrics and Gynaecology in the UK [77]. This also applies to most other specialties, in line with the recommendations of the Academy of Medical Royal Colleges and the NHS institute for Innovation and Improvement.

Nowhere is leadership more crucial to improving care quality than on the front line—in wards, clinics and general practices. Leadership at the front line is often best performed by clinicians (usually doctors and nurses), together with general managers. Frontline clinicians exercise considerable influence over staff and patients. What they say and what they do have a significant impact on those they lead, as they will be taken to be communicating the organisation's priorities and values [78]. Therefore all clinicians need to be competent managers and leaders in their practitioner roles. This is due to their direct and far-reaching impact on patient experience and outcomes and their broad legal duty, which means they have an intrinsic leadership role within healthcare services. It is also about the recognition that without doctors actively involved in the management, leadership and transformation of health services, initiatives to improve the patient experience are unlikely to succeed [79].

5.12 The Medical Leadership Competency Framework (MLCF)

In the UK a new leadership framework was recently introduced called the 'Healthcare Leadership Model'. This framework seeks to identify to what extent leaders have developed or are developing leadership behaviours within the nine leadership dimensions. This framework and others used across the globe, enable self reflection in three main areas: self awareness (an exploration of one's' strengths and limitations), the delivery of and improvement of services and strategy (setting direction). While there are numerous competency frameworks available, the general view is that it is not necessarily the version of the framework that is important, rather it is the focus on the act of reflection to identify areas for personal development. The Medical Leadership Competency Framework is another such framework that has been developed in the UK and will be recognisable to many doctors as the domains have become embedded in their post graduate medical curricula. The MLCF [80] (Fig. 5.4) developed by The Academy of Medical Royal Colleges and the NHS institute for Innovation and Improvement is the first leadership and management competency framework that is applicable to

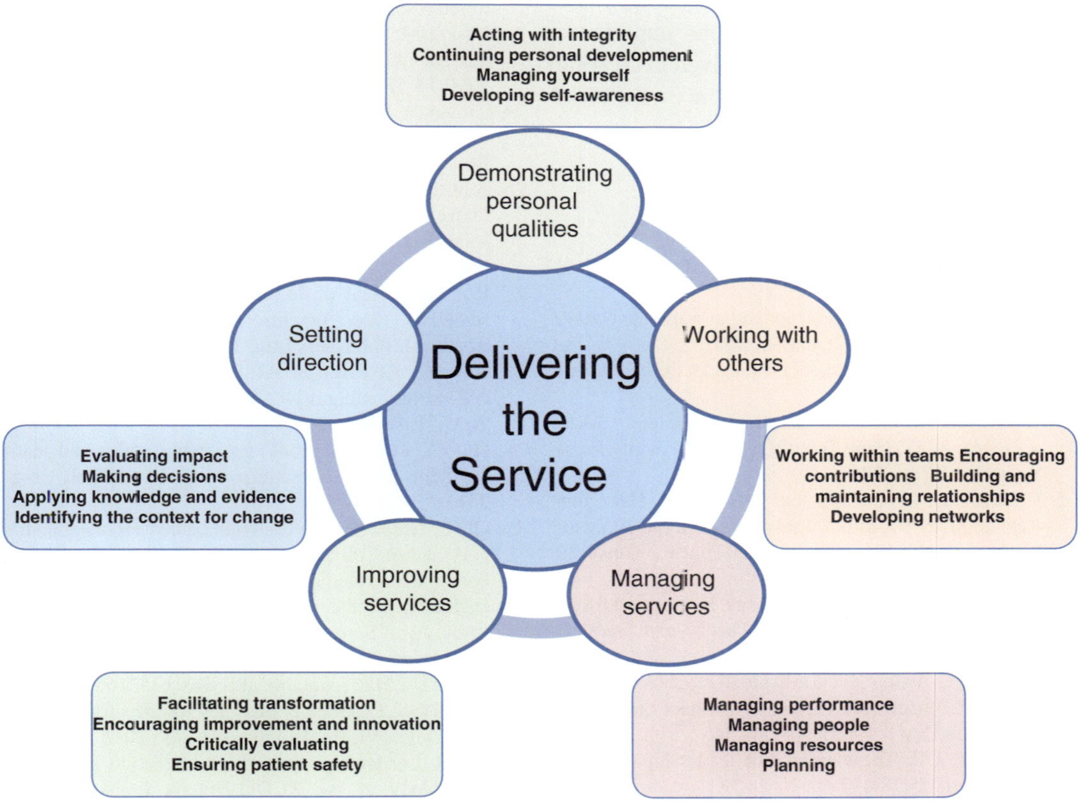

Fig. 5.4 Domains of medical leadership competency framework

all stages of a doctors training and career and in their practitioner roles. The MLCF describes 'the leadership competencies doctors need to become more actively involved in the planning, delivery and transformation of health services as a normal part of their role as doctors'. A significant aspect of the MLCF is that it is based on the concept of shared leadership 'where leadership is not restricted to people who hold designated leadership roles, and where there is a shared sense of responsibility for the success of the organisation and its services' [79]. There are five domains of the MLCF (Fig. 5.4) and it is considered essential that every doctor demonstrates competence in each domain to deliver appropriate, safe and effective services. Within each domain there are four elements and each of these elements is further divided into four competency outcomes. As the development of formal leadership and management competence becomes an integral part of doctors' training and learning, it will stimulate more doctors to take on service improvement and executive leadership roles. It will also encourage more non-clinical leaders to recognise the importance of real engagement and to be involved in creating cultures and incentives that value the contribution of all doctors [79].

References

1. Crainer S. The FT handbook of management. London: Pitman; 1995.
2. Mullins LJ. Management and organisational behaviour. Essex: Pearson Education; 2007.
3. Gill R. Theory and practice of leadership. London: Sage; 2011.
4. Hellriegel D, et al. Management: second South African edition. Cape Town: Oxford University Press Southern Africa; 2004.
5. Goleman D. Leadership that gets results. Harv Bus Rev. 2000:76–91. http://elibrary.kiu.ac.ug:8080/jspui/bitstream/1/480/1/Leadership%20That%20Gets%20Results.pdf
6. Swanepoel B, Erasmus B, Schenk H. South African human resource management. Theory and practice. Cape Town: Juta and Co. Ltd; 2008.
7. Bernard LL. An introduction to social psychology. 1926.
8. Hersey P, Blanchard KH. Life cycle theory of leadership. Train Dev J. 1969;23(5):26–34.
9. Kilbourne CE. The elements of leadership. J Coast Artillery. 1935;78:437–9.
10. Maude B. Leadership in management. London: Business Books; 1978.
11. Stogdill RM. Handbook of leadership: a survey of theory and research. Ney York: Free Press; 1974.
12. Senior B, Fleming J. Organizational change. Essex: Pearson Education; 2006.
13. Derue DS, et al. Trait and behavioural theories of leadership: an integration and meta-analytic test of their relative validity. Pers Psychol. 2011;64(1):7–52.
14. Epstein S. Trait theory as personality theory: can a part be as great as the whole? Psychol Inq. 1994;5(2):120–2.
15. Ayman R, Korabik K. Leadership: why gender and culture matter. Am Psychol. 2010;65(3):157.
16. Daft RL. Leadership: theory and practice: Harcourt College Pub.; 1999.
17. Shriberg A, Shriberg D, Lloyd CA. Practicing leadership: principles and applications. New York: Wiley; 2002.
18. McGregor D. The human side of enterprise, vol. 21. New York; 1960. p. 166.
19. Bass BM. Bass and Stogdill's handbook of leadership: theory, research and managerial applications. New York: Free Press; 1990.
20. Blake RR, Mouton JS. Management by Grid® principles or situationalism: which? Group Org Manag. 1981;6(4):439–55.
21. Bass BM. Transformational leadership: industrial, military, and educational impact. Mahwah: Lawrence Erlbaum and Associates; 1998.
22. Hersey, P., Blanchard, K.H. Management of organizational resources: utilising human resources. 1988.
23. Bass BM, Avolio BJ. Developing transformational leadership: 1992 and beyond. J Eur Ind Train. 1990;14(5):21–7.
24. Crossman A. Deductive reasoning versus inductive reasoning. 2013. http://sociology.about.com/od/Research/a/Deductive-Reasoning-Versus-Inductive-Reasoning.htm.
25. Johnson M. Managing in the next millennium. Oxford: Butterworth-Heinemann; 1995.
26. Johnson G, Whittington R, Scholes K. Exploring corporate strategy. 9th ed. Essex: FT Prentice Hall; 2011.
27. Robson C. Real world research: a resource for social scientists and practitioners-researchers. Oxford: Blackwell Publishers Ltd.; 1993.
28. Blom M, Alvesson M. All-inclusive and all good: the hegemonic ambiguity of leadership. Scand J Manag. 2015;31(4):480–92.
29. Hu YY, et al. Surgeons' leadership styles and team behavior in the operating room. J Am Coll Surg. 2016;222(1):41–51.
30. Ola B. Leadership styles: team behaviour or safer surgery? J Am Coll Surg. 2016;222(5):967.
31. Parker SH, Yule S, Flin R, McKinley A. Surgeons' leadership in the operating room: an observational study. Am J Surg. 2012;204(3):347–54.
32. Chendroyaperumal C. Theory of 'Great Leadership' is missing! 2011. Available at SSRN 1752166
33. Gujral GS. Leadership qualities for effective leaders. New Delhi: Vij Books India Pvt Ltd.; 2012.
34. Ola B. Leadership styles in global health initiatives: case study of the RCOG-Nigeria Liaison Group. MBA Dissertation, Sheffield Hallam University; Unpublished. 2016.

35. Bass BM, Avolio BJ. Multifactor leadership questionnaire. Redwood City: Mind Garden. 2000.
36. Yukl G. Leadership in organisations. Englewood Cliffs: Prentice-Hall; 1998.
37. Bass BM. Concepts of leadership. In: Vecchio RP, editor. Leadership: understanding the dynamics of power and influence in organizations. Notre Dame: University of Notre Dame Press; 1997.
38. Lagomarsino R, Cardona P. Relationships among leadership, organizational commitment in Uruguayan Health Business Studies and Institutions. No D/494 in IESE Research Papers from IESE Business School. 2003.
39. Mester C, Visser D, Roodt G. Leadership style and its relation to employee attitudes and behaviour. SA J Ind Psychol. 2003;29(2):72–80.
40. Burns JM. Leadership. New York: Harper and Row Publishers; 1978.
41. Avolio BJ, Waldman DA, Yammarino FJ. Leading in the 1990's: the four I's of transformational leadership. J Eur Ind Train. 1991;15:1–8.
42. Meyer M, Botha E. Organisation development and transformation in South Africa. Durban: Butterworths; 2000.
43. Bass BM, Avolio BJ. Transformational leadership development: manual for MLQ. Palo Alto: Consulting Psychologist Press; 1990.
44. Bolden R, et al. A review of leadership theory and competency frameworks. Centre for leadership studies, Exeter: University of Exeter; 2003.
45. Xirasagar S, Samuels ME, Stoskopf CH. Physician leadership styles and effectiveness: an empirical study. Med Care Res Rev. 2005;62(6):720–40.
46. Wolmarans S, Martins N. The 360 degree emotional competency profiler. Johannesburg: Organisational Diagnostics and Learning Link International; 2001. Unpublished manual
47. Martinez MN. The smarts that count. HR Magazine. 1997;42(11):72–8.
48. Goleman D. Leadership that gets results. Harvard Business Review Onpoint. Hbr.org; 2013. p. 26–38.
49. Thorndike EL. A constant error in psychological ratings. J Appl Psychol. 1920;4:25–9.
50. Gardner H. Frames of mind. New York: Bantam; 1983.
51. Gardner H, Hatch T. Multiple intelligences go to school. Educ Res. 1989;18(8):8–14.
52. Salovey P, Mayer JD. Emotional intelligence. Imagin Cogn Pers. 1990;9:185–211.
53. Mayer JD, Caruso D, Salovey P. Competing models of emotional intelligence. In: Steinberg RJ, editor. Handbook of human intelligence. 2nd ed. New York: Cambridge University Press; 1998.
54. Palmer B, et al. Emotional intelligence and effective leadership. Leadersh Org Dev J. 2001;22(20):1–7.
55. Bar-On R. Bar-On emotional quotient inventory technical manual. New York: Multi-Health Systems; 1997.
56. Bar-On R. Emotional and social intelligence. In: Bar-On R, JDA P, editors. The handbook of emotional intelligence. San Francisco: Jossey-Bass; 2000.
57. Wolmarans IS. Emotional competencies of the future. Johannesburg: Learning Link International; 2001. Unpublished paper
58. Palmer PN, Jansen CA, Coetzee M. Perceptions of South African managers' emotional intelligence: a preliminary investigation. SA Bus Rev. 2006;10(1):91–110.
59. Theron D, Roodt G. An evaluation of the 360° project management competency assessment questionnaire. SA J Ind Psychol. 2001;27(2):51–6.
60. Schutte NS, et al. Development and validation of a measure of emotional intelligence. Personal Individ Differ. 1998;25:167–77.
61. Huy QN. Emotional capability, emotional intelligence, and radical change. Acad Manag Rev. 1999;24(2):325–45.
62. Dulewicz V, Higgs M. Emotional intelligence—a review and evaluation study. J Manag Psychol. 2000;15(4):341–72.
63. Kelley R, Caplan J. How Bell Labs creates star performers. Harv Bus Rev. 1993;3(2):100–3.
64. Faiz O, et al. Is theatre utilization a valid performance indicator for NHS operating theatres? BMC Health Serv Res. 2008;8:28. doi:10.1186/1472-6963-8-28.
65. Amos TL, Ristow A, Ristow L. Human resource management. 2nd ed. Lansdowne: Juta; 2004.
66. Kaplan RS, Norton DP. The balance scorecard. Boston: The Harvard Business School Press; 1996.
67. Kaplan RS. Strategic performance measurement and management in non-profit organizations. Non-Profit Manage Leadersh. 2001;11(3):353–70.
68. Bass BM, Avolio BJ. Transformational leadership: a response to critics. In: Leadership theory and research: perspectives and directions; 1993. p. 49–80.
69. Pruijn GHJ, Boucher RL. The relationship of transactional and transformational leadership to the organisational effectiveness of the dutch national sports organisations. Eur J Sports Manage. 1994;1:72–87.
70. Brand C, Heyl G, Maritz D. Leadership. In: Meyer M, Botha E, editors. Organisational development and transformation in South Africa. Durban: Butterworths; 2000.
71. Haygroup. Leadership and talent. 2013. Available at: http://www.haygroup.com/ww/services/index.aspx?id=104
72. Keogh T, Martin WM. Managing unmanageable physicians: leadership, stewardship, and disruptive behavior. Physician Exec. 2004;30(5):18–23.
73. Schwartz RW, Tumblin TF. The power of servant leadership to transform health care organizations for the 21st-century economy. Arch Surg. 2002;137(12):1419.
74. Catano VM, Pond M, Kelloway EK. Exploring commitment and leadership in volunteer organisations. Leadersh Org Dev J. 2001;22(6):256–63.
75. Hind P, Wilson A, Lenssen G. Developing leaders for sustainable business. Corp Gov. 2009;9(1):7–20.
76. Clark J. Medical leadership and engagement: no longer an optional extra. J Health Organ Manag. 2012;26(4):437–43.
77. RCOG. Educational progress matrix ST1 to ST7 for 2014–15. 2016. https://www.rcog.org.uk/globalassets/documents/careers-and-training/assessment-and-progression-through-training/training_matrix.pdf.

78. The King's Fund. Patient-centred leadership: rediscovering our purpose. London: Kings Fund; 2013. Available at: http://www.kingsfund.org.uk/publications/patient-centred-leadership
79. Clark J, Armit K. Leadership competency for doctors: a framework. Leadersh Health Serv. 2010;23(2):115–29. Available at: http://www.emeraldinsight.com/doi/full/10.1108/17511871011040706
80. NHS Institute for Innovation and Improvement and Academy of Medical Royal Colleges. Medical leadership competency framework. 2nd ed. Coventry: NHS Institute for Innovation and Improvement; 2009.
81. Bass BM, Avolio BJ. Improving organisational effectiveness through transformational leadership. London: Sage; 1994

6 Effective Hospital Leadership: Theory and Practice

Simon Boyes and Jill Aylott

The Kirkup Report (2015) found that there were 20 instances of significant or major failure of care at the Furness General Hospital (FGH) in the UK, associated with three maternal deaths and 16 deaths of babies at or after birth. The report ruled that there was a *"seriously dysfunctional nature of the maternity service at FGH, with clinical competence substandard, with deficit skills and knowledge"* ([1], p. 7). Simply employing health professionals in roles that define a level of professional competence and confirm a 'scope of practice' within a regulatory health care body, will not be enough to ensure patient safety. While interprofessional practice and multi-disciplinary team working is promoted as best practice in health care, in reality there are professional boundary disputes and contested professional territories [2–4]. It is evident that professionals will use a form of professional rhetoric in the name of "patient centred" and "holistic care" as a bid to support legitimacy in claiming role exclusivity or at least primacy in an aspect of health care [2]. At the FGH, there was a failure to be open and honest with patients and relatives while midwives, obstetricians and paediatricians failed to work together which resulted in "midwives pursuing normal childbirth at any cost", without being challenged, which resulted in a "dysfunctional nature of professional relationships" ([1], p. 7).

The executive managers of a hospital need to be reassured that the healthcare workforce is not only clinically competent to deliver safe and effective services to patients, but to be equally reassured that there is standardisation in non-clinical competencies in leadership and management and quality improvement. More integration of clinical competence with leadership and management is required and one example of an integrated competency framework is a new competency based MBA for health professionals based on the model developed by Camuffo and Gerli [5]. Adding to this complexity is a continued shortage of specific specialties in medicine, nursing and AHPs which presents the dual challenge of professionals seeking more autonomy in practice to defend their professional role [1, 2, 6] while placing healthcare systems under extreme pressure resulting in the closure of some services and depleted resources in others.

Never before has there been such a need for an investment in an innovative and creative solution to the global healthcare workforce crisis. This chapter will outline the complex context of the policy changes affecting the employment of drs in healthcare in the UK and argue that a future workforce solution must include the development of

S. Boyes (✉)
Sheffield Teaching Hospitals NHS Foundation Trust, Sheffield, UK
e-mail: Simon.Boyes@sth.nhs.uk

J. Aylott
Directorate for International MBA Programmes, International Academy of Medical Leadership, Sheffield, UK
e-mail: Jill.Aylott@iamedicalleadership.com

P. Godbole et al. (eds.), *Why Hospitals Fail*, DOI 10.1007/978-3-319-56224-7_6

core international healthcare competencies that define the delivery of quality of care for patients [7]. Such a solution requires hospitals to dedicate an investment of time within a model of 'invest to save'. Without the time of key stakeholders being accounted for away from delivering clinical activity, such a solution simply will not happen.

6.1 Increased Demand and Limited Resources

In the UK there have been several changes since 1999 that have had significant implications on the provision of 24 h 7 days a week medical and surgical coverage of inpatients and emergency admissions. These are detailed below.

6.2 New Deal and European Working Time Directive (EWTD)

Before the introduction of the new deal and EWTD the majority of medical staff when on call would work 24–32 h on weekdays and up to 72 h on a weekend. In 1991 the new deal for doctors was introduced to make significant improvements in the working hours and life for junior doctors. The new deal stipulated a maximum number of hours worked, maximum continuous duty period, minimum rest during duty periods and minimum period off duty between duty periods which would vary depending on whether it was a full, partial or on call rota [8].

In 1993 the EWTD was introduced, the aim was to limit the time spent at work in order to protect workers health and safety [9]. It wasn't until 1998 that the EWTD was introduced for consultants limiting their working week to 48 h though there is the option to opt out to a limit of 56 h [10]. The EWTD for junior doctors had a staggered introduction with full implementation being in August 2009 again with a voluntary opt out of 56 h [11]. Part of this legislation introduced the requirement for a minimum 11 h rest period in every 24 h. Two rulings by the European Court of Justice the SIMAP in 2000 and Jaeger in 2003 stated that for the full period of time a doctor was in their place of work even if sleeping should be counted as work [12].

These two pieces of legislation and subsequent rulings have had significant implications for the provision of compliant rotas. For a rota to be compliant it has to be a full shift rota except in a few low intensity specialities where it is still possible to have a 24 h non resident on call rota. This has required an increase in the number of junior doctors required to adequately fill the rota as well as give continued protection for job related training. In 2014 there were 53,786 whole time equivalent (WTE) doctors in training compared to 33,932 in 2002. In the same period consultant numbers also rose by 3.4% per year from 24,756 to 40,443 WTE [13]. For those organisations that don't provide a EWTD compliant rota it has financial implications. The Health and Safety Executive can impose fines for any breaches (£5000 per employee per breach) and non compliant post attract a 100% supplement for out of hours work calculated as a proportion of the basic salary compared to the 20–50% supplement for compliant rotas [14].

In 2016 a new contract for doctors in training was negotiated by the NHS employers and the British Medical Association (BMA) this has been imposed following its rejection by the BMA membership. This has removed the banding supplements but can result in significant penalties for hours worked over those specified in the rota. Through the provision of work schedules there is an improved recognition of the training requirements for an individual and if these are not achieved can be raised as for hours worked over as an exception report. The aim is that the training opportunity is then made available to the trainee. This rightly recognises the training element of training posts but brings into sharp focus the implications on the delivery of the routine work required for patient care.

6.3 Changing Face of Specialist Training

In the last 20 years there have been several changes in the way postgraduate medical training is delivered. In 1993, The Calman Report, Hospitals Doctors-Training for the Future recommended a reduction of the minimum length of specialist training to 7 years, the award of a certificate of completion of specialist training by the General Medical Council, completing a structured training curriculum and merging the registrar and senior registrar grades [15].

In 2002, the Chief Medical Officer published Unfinished Business which was an attempt to address the deficiencies in the senior house officer grade of which 50% were in service posts rather than training the so called lost tribe [16]. It also had implications for specialist training and for non consultant career grade doctors giving the chance to enter or re-enter specialist training. Following consultation these changes to training were enshrined in Modernising Medical Careers-The Next Steps [17]. In 2005 the changes were introduced with a 2 year foundation programme following graduation with entry on to a run through 7 year specialist training programme via a centralised selection process starting in 2007, which would lead to a certificate of completion of training.

Due to major failings in the centralised selection process (Medical Training Application Service (MTAS)) in 2007, the Department of Health announced an independent inquiry into Modernising Medical Careers (MMC) which was chaired by Professor Sir John Tooke and his recommendation were published in his final report Aspiring to Excellence [18]. The DOH published its final response to the recommendations Implementing the Tooke Report: Department of Health Update [19] which resulted in changes to the delivery of medical training. Minor changes to the structure of the training programmes were implemented with selection occurring following the foundation programme for core speciality training (2 years) and prior to speciality training (5–6 years).

In October 2015 following on from the independent shape of training review the Royal College of Surgeons released the Improving Surgical Training (IST) report which made 26 recommendations for changes in surgical training [20, 21]. In conjunction with Health Education England the aim is to pilot these changes to training in general surgery. This will be competency based training rather than time served with a greater shift in the balance towards training rather than service. Implications are that there will be a move to rotas that allow a greater proportion of day time training and a greater role for simulation. There was recognition that there will be a requirement for other professionals to deliver patient care to allow time for this training.

6.4 Eligibility for Specialist Training

The NHS plan, A plan for investment, A plan for reform [22] had set out moves to make the UK self sufficient for its medical workforce needs. This required increasing the number of medical school places following recommendations by the Medical Workforce Standing Advisory Committee [23]. Due to a significant shortfall in medical human resource, there had been a mechanism where non European economic area (EAA) medical graduates were able to work and train in the UK permit free. In April 2006 the Home Office announced that it was going to end permit free training [24]. From 2009, Non EAA doctors are no longer eligible to apply for a speciality training programme [24]. Previously Non EAA doctors would take up non training posts in the UK as they saw it as a stepping stone on to speciality training. This is no longer an option and discourages their application for such posts though they are eligible with a Tier 2 visa. In February 2013, nationally there were 325 WTE training posts that were filled by locums [25].

6.5 Case Study: Workforce Planning and the Renal Surgery Rota

Following the impending implementation of the EWTD it was not feasible for renal surgery to provide a EWTD compliant rota in isolation. Renal surgery middle grade cover in 2008 was provided by two Speciality grade doctors and a research fellow. Funding was sought from the Strategic Health Authority for an additional renal surgery post with the aim of providing input into the general surgery rota. In 2009, this new clinical fellow post and two other posts from renal surgery became part of the general surgery rota with an agreed cross cover arrangements at night and weekends for renal surgery.

6.6 Recruitment Issues

In 2012 the research fellow and one of the speciality doctors resigned leaving a gap in the rota. The speciality doctor post has subsequently been filled but this was by the incumbent clinical fellow who was the only applicant for the post. The clinical fellow post has been readvertised on two separate occasions with no suitable or no applicants this is similar to the pattern for all middle grade posts advertised in renal surgery since 2008. The consequence has been that the rota gaps have been filled by locums at a cost for 2012/13 of £191,040.

6.7 General Surgery Rota

The general surgery rota was populated by 3 renal surgery posts, 2 general surgery speciality doctors and 13 specialist registrars. From October 2013 there was increasing pressure on the rota due to changes in training requirements. Vascular surgery in 2013 became recognised as a speciality in its own right and therefore trainees no longer need to take part in the general surgery rota. In addition final year sub speciality trainees in breast and endocrine with the approval of the Training Programme Director do not have to be part of the general surgery rota.

6.8 Hospital at Night

August 2011 saw the introduction of Hospital at Night (H@N) which was originally proposed as a way of reducing the dependency on training grade doctors in dealing with healthcare needs of patients out of hours. The approach uses a multidisciplinary team, with a dedicated handover period and strict bleep policy. This level of coordination means that on call medical staff can be directed to those patients that require specialist expertise with other problems being dealt with by highly skilled trained nurse practitioners. The original pilots were started in four trusts in 2004 and an evaluation report demonstrated that H@N helped improve patient care and had no negative impact on doctors training [26]. In 2013/14 and 2014/15 there was a reduction in the number of training post at foundation level with four posts being lost locally. H@N has been able to provide sufficient support to cover the gaps in the rota due to these reductions. H@N besides helping with the intensity of the middle grade workload at night it cannot compensate for any loss in human resource at this grade.

6.9 PESTEL Framework

The PESTEL framework will help summarise the macro environmental factors that impact on the organisation ability to deal with workforce issues and help identify the key drivers of change ([27], p. 50).

Political	Technological
• Changes to visa requirements • Adoption of EWTD and new deal • Changes to speciality training • Contract changes • Changes to retirement age • No more money for the NHS	• Information Technology • Communications • New ways of working (telemedicine)
Economic	**Environmental**
• Locum costs for rota gaps • Financial cost of non compliant rota (corporate risk) • Skill shortages • Changing skill mix • Cost improvement programmes • "Nicholson Challenge"	• Increased community care • Increase in day case procedures
Social	**Legislation**
• Employee expectations (work life balance) • Education and Training • Flexible working opportunities • Unpopular Speciality • Non training post • Changing demographic • Patient expectations	• SIMAP and Jaeger rulings • EWTD • New Deal • Health and Safety legislation

6.10 Key Drivers for Change

The situation of continuing to support the renal and general surgery rota gaps was financially unsustainable with the high locum costs involved and the continued difficulty in recruiting to a substantive post. Withdrawing two renal posts from the rota in addition to the other pressures on the rota would have a significant impact on the training and education of the specialist registrars. The current skill mix does not allow for the amelioration of the effect of reducing the numbers populating the general surgery rota. Any changes will need to be in line with the directorates cost improvement plan of 2 to 5% per annum and depending on the current spending review this maybe on going to 2020.

6.11 Vision

To develop a long term sustainable cost effective workforce strategy for renal surgery whilst improving the quality of the service and minimising the impact on the education and training of the general surgery specialist registrars.

6.12 Strategic Options

There are two options that may achieve the above vision and each merits consideration. Each of the options will be described and to evaluate the best strategy for the organisation, Johnson et al have described three criteria that determine the potential success of any particular strategic option. These criteria using the acronym SAFe are:

- Suitability does the strategy use the organisations strengths or opportunities and avoid any weaknesses or threats.
- Acceptability does it meet the expectation of its stakeholders
- Feasibility would a proposed strategy work in practice

([27], p. 363)

6.13 Improving Acceptability of Current Posts (Option 1)

This option would be to look at the current unfilled posts and identify the factors that would make them more attractive to applicants. The ideal scenario would be for the post to be assigned a national training number and therefore be recognised as a training post for renal transplantation. An alternative would be to look at the post having greater cross speciality integration with general surgery which may increase its acceptability.

The other post was a research post in conjunction with the local University. To provide a salary, the incumbent had a service commitment to renal and general surgery. With the right research programme the post could be attractive to speciality registrars looking for 1–2 years out of programme experience leading to a higher research degree. The alternative is to look at the feasibility in converting this post to full time service post which covers both renal and general surgery.

6.14 Advanced Nurse Practitioner (ANP), Surgical Care Practitioners (SCP) or Physician Associate/ Assistant (PA) (Option 2)

The development of the role of the Advanced Nurse Practitioner (ANP) has a long history with the first nurse practitioner programme appearing in the USA in 1965 [28]. ANP are nurses who have expanded and extended their roles to be able to diagnose and treat a wide range of clinical conditions beyond that attained at their initial registration. The NHS plan highlighted that there had to be significant changes to the "*old demarcations*" and that the development of suitability qualified nurses to be able perform a wider range of clinical tasks should be encouraged [22]. There had been for long periods an inconsistent approach to what was defined as advanced practice for nurses. The Department of Health published Advanced Level Nursing-A Position Statement which helped resolve these inconsistencies [29]. The Royal College of Nursing have documented the level of practice and competencies that define the role of the ANP and specified that in the future this should be at masters level [30]. The quality and outcomes of care provided by ANPs has been shown to be at least equivalent to that provided by doctors [31, 32].

A further addition to these roles has been the development of the Surgical Care Practitioner (SCP) who in addition to providing clinical care for patients also assists in the operating theatre. If they are suitably trained they also may perform certain surgical procedures including wound opening/closure, vein harvesting, and catheterisation. A working party including the Royal College of Surgeons of England and the National Practitioners Programme have produced The Curriculum Framework for the Surgical Care Practitioner which has laid out an educational programme, competencies and standards required to work as an SCP [33] and a subsequent revision was published in 2014 [34]. The curriculum covers several surgical specialities but not one that is specific to renal surgery however the core requirements are covered under general, vascular and cardiothoracic surgery. The SCP can not only be drawn from qualified nurses but also those trained as operating department practitioners.

PAs are biomedical science graduates who after completing a 2 year postgraduate diploma can then work in a healthcare setting. In 2006 the DOH published The Curriculum and Competency Framework for Physicians Assistant in conjunction with the Royal Colleges of Physicians and General Practitioners with a subsequent revision in 2012 with the additional involvement of the Royal Colleges of Surgeons and Emergency Medicine [33, 34, 35]. The PA model was originally developed in the United States of America in the 1960s to provide healthcare to under resourced areas but it wasn't until 2003 that they first made an appearance in the UK working within primary care [36]. The role of PA is not statutory regulated though to add assurance around public protection and safety in 2010 the PA Voluntary Managed Registrar was established and is now administered by the newly formed Faculty of Physicians Associates under the auspice of the Royal College of Physicians (England). To be maintained on the register the PA have to undergo a process of recertification every 6 years though due to the lack of statutory regulation it is not currently mandatory to be registered. Unlike ANPs and SCPs the limitation of the PA role is that they currently cannot prescribe and as the requesting of radiological examination involves the prescribing of ionising radiation they are unable to request these tests. The GMC view is that for PAs to prescribe will require statutory regulation but they have not specified whether that's by them or another body [37].

This option would involve converting the current unfilled posts into two ANP, SCP or PA roles but this would result in renal surgery not being able to populate two slots on the general surgery on call rota. It would however provide sustainable service provision to the renal surgery service. Due to the lack of non-medical prescribing a requirement for this role PAs will not be considered further. These two options will be evaluated together using the SAFe framework with ANP being interchangeable with SCP.

6.15 Suitability

From reviewing the PESTEL analysis it follows that the first option will continue to maintain the status quo and reduce the risks of the general surgery rota not being able to meet the demands of the EWTD. The change of role to ANPs and the other threats to the numbers populating the general surgery rota will put significant strain on the rota if it continues in the current format. The main weakness would be the difficulty in maintaining the education and training value of the general surgery posts as there would be an increase in the frequency of the emergency component of the post.

From the economic perspective both options would potentially reduce the need for employing locums to fill the renal surgery post with a significant reduction in ongoing locum costs but with a higher likelihood of continuity in the ANP posts. The weakness of option 1 is that it is dependent on being able to facilitate an ongoing fully funded research programme which allows for service commitment and being able to attract the appropriate applicants. Option 1 would be continuing the commitment to general surgery and therefore an ongoing risk if no suitable post holders of ongoing locum costs. The other weakness of option 1, even with making the post a more attractive non training post there is likely to be periods when the post will remain unfilled. If the post got recognition as a renal transplant training post there still wouldn't be any guarantee that the post would be filled on a yearly basis as there are a limited number of trainees.

The strength of the ANP option is that the organisation already has significant experience in using ANPs in the acute care setting both in H@N, the emergency department and the cardiothoracic unit. The model used in the cardiothoracic unit is the approach that renal surgery would adopt. The weakness is the lead time of 18–24 months required to train an ANP to become autonomous in the role.

6.16 Acceptability

6.16.1 Cost Analysis

On starting the post ANP are initially paid at band 6 of the agenda for change the top of the scale being £34,350. Additional costs to the department would be the cost of training to achieve the appropriate competencies. A part time postgraduate diploma in surgical care practice from an accredited University has average annual fees of £4600 a year. There would also be the requirement to provide some locum medical cover during this 18 month training period when annual leave and on call commitments of the Speciality grade doctors coincide. With careful planning the level of this additional cost could be ameliorated but would equate to £1416/week (40 h at £35.40/hr (capped rates April 2016). On completion of training they move to band 7, top of the scale would be £40,558. Further salary uplift would be an additional £7000 for on-call or out of hour's commitments giving a full salary on achieving the top of the scale of £47,558 [38].

The renal surgery post is unlikely to attract anyone with seniority greater than speciality registrar six especially if this was a training post the salary range would be £35,592 to £41,564. The post is banded at 1b attracting a supplement of 40% which equates to a range of £14,236 to £16,625. The full salary range is £49,828 to £58,189. This does not take into account the potential need to fill gaps in medical cover with locums, the cost for a 6 month period would approximate to £59,800 [39]. The salary costs do not take into account the employer on costs for pension contributions, national insurance etc.

Even with potential additional cost pressure to renal surgery in the ANP training period it can be seen that ANPs are cost effective in comparison to the continued use of medical staff.

6.17 Stakeholders

From the perspective of the stakeholders in general surgery and renal surgery the preferred option would be to have a sustainable medical workforce as proposed in option one. The surgical trainees in general surgery are finding that the current rota is having an affect on their training. The reduction in the numbers on the rota by potentially up to five would still keep the rota as EWTD compliant but would reduce the number of weeks on elective activity by a quarter not taking into account the affect of annual and study leave. A change in the rota removing the second on registrar would only gain 4 weeks of elective activity per year but may have significant affect on quality and safety of the care received by patients admitted as emergencies. The converse is also true that there are significant governance issues with reduced availability of registrars being able to provide senior cover to the inpatients. The resolution of these issues needs a rethink on how medical care is delivered in general surgery in hospitals in the future.

There is a knock on affect from the reduced numbers on the rota within renal surgery. One of the speciality doctors takes part in the rota and the change in on call frequency would reduce his elective activity in renal surgery. The speciality doctors provide cross cover for clinics and operating list when consultants are not available and so may result in renal surgery being unable to cover profiled lists with the loss of income.

The funding for the current posts is provided via the renal directorate budget which renal surgery is a small part. The current situation is not sustainable in light of the high locum costs and the feeling within the directorate is that a long term solution has to be achieved. The ANP/SCP option is likely to offer the most sustainable cost effective solution to the medical staffing issues within renal surgery and potentially could offer savings towards the directorates cost improvement programme.

6.18 Feasibility

Renal surgery currently performs around 60 transplants per year, with the growth in organ donor numbers and allocation changes this number should potentially increase year on year. The minimum number of transplants to attract a national training number is 72 transplants per year in the short term this will not be consistently achievable. In addition to this the Centre for Workforce Intelligence has recommended the reduction in the NTNs for speciality registrars from 158 to 123 per year in general surgery which transplant is part of [40]. The current posts are therefore likely to remain as non training posts even with changes to make the post more attractive are unlikely to attract suitable candidates especially with continuing visa restrictions. The lead time for setting up and funding a research programme will be a minimum of a year. Doubts must remain that such an appropriately funded programme would allow the research fellow time to provide a service commitment to renal and general surgery.

The funding stream currently used to support the current unfilled posts could be used to fund two ANP or SCP plus their training. Other source of funding for the training element could be sought from trust funds if there is an unlikely shortfall. Certain aspects of the service would need a rethink on how it is delivered whilst the ANPs were in training. This would mostly be related to the assessment of acute renal surgical problems but with appropriate protocols and support arrangements should be achievable using current resources.

6.19 The Future Healthcare Workforce: A Competency Based Approach

With evidence that contested professional boundaries in healthcare is alive and flourishing [2], the growth of new roles in surgery must learn from the "dysfunctional nature of professional relationships" that existed at Morcambe Bay hospital [1]. While the SCP curriculum is competency based, there is scope for the enhancement and development of the competency based approach to embrace all professionals within a field of healthcare practice.

A competency is defined as a capability or ability. It is a set of related but different sets of behaviour organised around an underlying construct which is called 'intent' [41]. Boyzatis provides an example of a competence in listening, he argues that listening can be demonstrated at two levels: a person could ask questions of a person to ingratiate themselves with a person and appear interested in them or they could ask questions to listen to someone because he or she is interested in understanding the other person, his or her priorities or thoughts in a situation. The latter is called a demonstration of empathy and the underlying intent is to understand the person. Boyzatis argues that the underlying intent is a more subtle competency and is a form of emotional self awareness. Self awareness is self insight and self understanding. A competency calls for both action (a set of alternative behaviours) and 'intent' which calls for measurement and methods that allow for the assessment of both the presence of the behaviour and the influence of intent.

A theory of performance is the basis for the concept of competency and in the competency approach it is supported by a basic 'contingency theory'. "Maximum performance is believed to occur when the person's capability or talent is consistent with the needs of the job demands and the organisational environment [42, 43].

We can take the competencies required for the Renal Surgical rota and list them as follows

- Surgical care practitioner
  - First Assistant
    - Male and female catheterisation
    - Prepping and draping
    - Wound Closure

    - Drain insertion
  - Flexible cystoscopy
  - Live donor kidney perfusion
- Urgent and non urgent Access reviews (ward/outpatients)
  - Initial assessment
  - Arrange X-rays/scans/blood test
  - Arrange admission/outpatient follow up
  - Arrange theatre/radiological intervention
  - Non medical prescribing
- Outpatient follow up
  - Access
  - Transplant
- On Call
  - Weekends when Transplant/GS on call
  - Not enough ANP for any other cover
  - Max 1:4

The above competencies would be classified as Tier 5 'industry specific' competencies. However in addition to this set of competencies there will need to be management and leadership competencies integrated with the clinical competencies as well as those from Tiers 1 to 3:

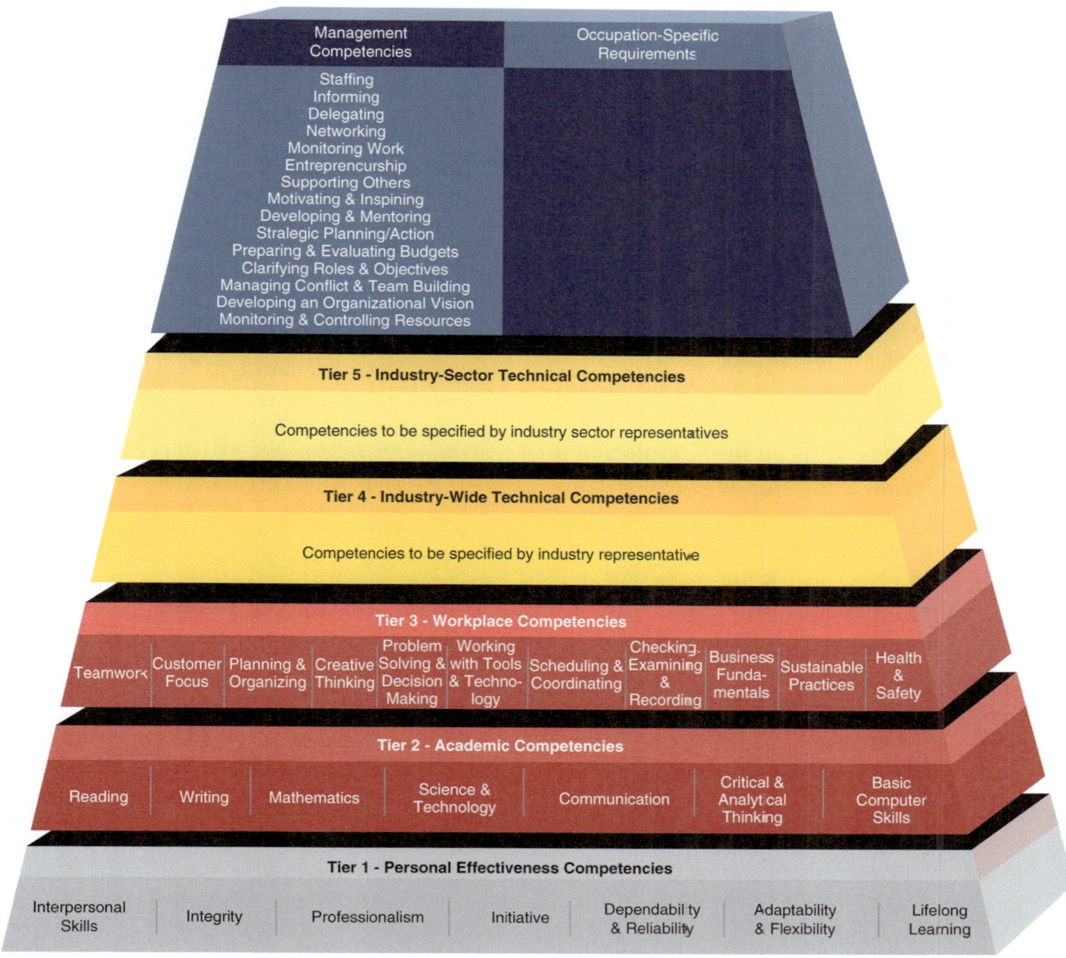

6.19.1 An Integrated Competency Framework

To develop a way forward and to gather a consensus on the level, type and amount of competencies, a survey can be sent out to key stakeholders to survey their views in the identification of the core competencies in this role. A similar process has been undertaken by Camuffo and Gerli [5] who set out to explore the requirements for an integrated competency based MBA. The authors used two surveys: the first was a management skills profile with 60 skills clustered into 12 areas and the executive skills profile of 48 skills split into 12 groups [44, 45]. The questions were asked how important each skill is perceived to be. Responses can be graded on a 7 point Likert scale. A competency framework can be used as a self assessment tool by potential applicant ANPs/SCP who are interested in undertaking the role while completing their training. The competency framework enables reassurance of the behaviour and the behavioural intent in this role.

6.19.2 Commitment to Develop Competency Frameworks

The development of a competent workforce in healthcare is well overdue as the tension continues between the defence of the profession and the changing needs of the population. Hospitals are clearly focussed on the operationalisation of the delivery of activity but investment of creative and innovative solutions is required urgently now to explore the deployment of a skilled healthcare workforce. Managers and Executives need to support medical leaders to spend time developing a workforce solution. Any time invested in non-clinical delivery will need the hospital executive sign off to a business case that recognises that the development of competency frameworks will take time to develop. This approach can only be advanced if there is commitment from the hospital executive to support this initiative as an 'invest to save' programme which will reap returns in time.

References

1. Kirkup B. The report of the Morcambe Bay investigation, 2015. www.gov.uk/government/publications.
2. King O, Nancarrow SA, Borthwick AM, Grace S. Contested professional role boundaries in health care: a systematic review of the literature. J Foot Ankle Res. 2015;8:2.
3. Nancarrow SA, Borthwick AM. Dynamic professional boundaries in the healthcare workforce. Sociol Health Med. 2005;27(1):897–919.
4. Timmons S, Tanner J. A disrupted occupational boundary: operating theatre nurses and operating department practitioners. Sociol Health Illn. 2004;26:645–66.
5. Camuffo A, Gerli F. An integrated competency based approach to management education an Italian MBA Case Study. Int J Train Dev. 2004;8(4):240–57.
6. Salhani D, Coulter I. The politics of interprofessional working and the struggle for professional autonomy in nursing. Soc Sci Med. 2009;68(7):1221–8.
7. Czabanowska K, Klemenc-Ketis Z, Potter A, Rochfort A, Tomasik T, Csiszar J, Van den Bussche P. Development of a competency framework for quality improvement in family medicine: a qualitative study. The Alliance for Continuing Education in the Health Professions, the Society for Academic Continuing Medical Education and the Council on CME, Association for Hospital Medical Education; 2012.
8. Executive NH. Junior Doctors: The new deal. Making the best use of skills of nurses and midwives. London: NHS Executive. 1991.
9. The Council of the European Union. Council directive 93/104/EC Brussels; 1993.
10. NHS Management Executive. Agreement by the joint negotiating committee (seniors) the working time directive implementation of the working time regulations. London: Department of Health; 1998.
11. Department of Health. A guide to the implications of the European Working Time Directive for doctors in training. London: Department of Health; 2009.
12. European Union Committee. European Union-ninth report. London: House of Lords; 2004. (9th)
13. Health and Social Care Information Centre. NHS Workforce Statistics in England, Summary of staff in the NHS - 2004–2014, Overview. 2015 [online]. Last accessed Nov 2016 at: http://content.digital.nhs.uk/catalogue/PUB16973/nhs-staf-2004-2014-over-rep.pdf.
14. NHS Employers. Working time directive 2009 frequently asked questions for trust implementation teams. London: NHS Confederation Company LTD; 2009.
15. Department of Health. Hospital doctors: training for the future. the report of the working group on specialist medical training. London: Department of Health; 1993.
16. Department of Health. Unfinished business proposals for reform of the senior house officer grade. A report by Sir Liam Donaldson Chief Medical Officer for England. A paper for consultation. London: Department of Health; 2002.
17. Department of Health. Modernising medical careers the next steps the future shape of foundation, specialist and general practice training programmes. London: Department of Health; 2004.
18. Health Education England. Aspiring to excellence: final report of the independent inquiry into modernising medical careers. London: Health Education England; 2008.
19. Department of Health. Implementing the tooke report: department of health update. London: Department of Health; 2008.
20. Greenaway D. Shape of training: securing the future of excellent patient care. Final report of the independent review led by professor david greenaway. General

medical council; 2013. http://www.shapeoftraining.co.uk/static/documents/content/Shape_of_training_FINAL_Report.pdf_53977887.pdf.
21. The Royal College of Surgeons of England. RCS professional standards improving surgical training. Proposal for a pilot surgical training programme. London: The Royal College of Surgeons of England; 2015. https://www.rcseng.ac.uk/-/media/files/rcs/careers-insurgery/improving_surgical_training_text.pdf.
22. Department of Health. The NHS plan. A plan for investment. A plan for reform. London: Department of Health; 2000.
23. Department of Health. Medical workforce standing advisory committee planning the medical workforce third report. London: Department of Health; 1997.
24. House of Commons Health Committee. Modernising medical careers third report of session 2007–08. London: Stationary Office; 2008. (3)
25. Health and Social Care Information Centre. NHS hospital and community health service (HCHS) workforce statistics in England, medical and dental staff – 2002–2012, as at 30 September, 2013. [online]. Last Accessed O6Jan 2013 at: http://www.hscic.gov.uk/searchcatalogue?productid=11217&topics=1%2fWorkforce%2fStaff+numbers&sort=Relevance&size=10&page=1#top.
26. Department of Health. The implementation and impact of hospital at night pilot projects an evaluation report. London: Department of Health; 2005.
27. Johnson G, Whittington R, Scholes K. Exploring strategy. Harlow: Pearson Education; 2011.
28. Dunn L. A literature review of advanced clinical nursing practice in the United States of America. J Adv Nurs. 1997;**25**(4):814–9.
29. Department of Health. Advanced level nursing: a position statement. London: Department of Health; 2010.
30. Royal College of Nursing. Advanced nurse practitioners – an RCN guide to advanced nursing practice, advanced nurse practitioners and programme accreditation. London: Royal College of Nursing; 2012.
31. O'Grady ET. Advanced practice registered nurses: the impact on patient safety and quality. In: Hughes RG, editor. Rockville: Agency for Healthcare Research and Quality, 2; 2008. p. 601–20.
32. Horrocks S. Systematic review of whether nurse practitioners working in primary care can provide equivalent care to doctors. BMJ. 2002;324(7341):819–23.
33. Department of Health. The curriculum framework for the surgical care practitioner. London: Department of Health; 2006.
34. RCSEng. The curriculum framework for the surgical care practitioner. London: The Royal College of Surgeons of England; 2014. http://accreditation.rcseng.ac.uk/pdf/SCP%20Curriculum%20Framework%202014.pdf. Accessed Nov 2016.
35. Department of Health. The competence and curriculum framework for the physician assistant. London: Department of Health; 2006. http://webarchive.nationalarchives.gov.uk/20130107105354/http://www.dh.gov.uk/prod_consum_dh/groups/dh_digitalassets/@dh/@en/documents/digitalasset/dh_4139319.pdf. Accessed Nov 2016.
36. P.A.M.V.R. Competence and curriculum framework for the physician assistant. London: Physician Assistant Managed Voluntary Register; 2012. https://static1.squarespace.com/static/544f552de4b0645de79fbe01/t/557f1c1ae4b0edab35dd92cf/1434393626361/CCF-27-03-12-for-PAMVR.pdf. Accessed Nov 2016.
37. Stewart A, Catanzaro R. Can physician assistants be effective in the UK? Clin Med. 2005;5(4):344–8.
38. NHS Employers. Pay circular (M&D) 1/2013. London: NHS Employers; 2013.
39. NHS Employers. Pay circular (AforC) 1/2013. London: NHS employers; 2013.
40. Centre for Workforce Intelligence. Medical specialty workforce summary sheet general surgery. London: Centre for Workforce Intelligence; 2011.
41. Boyzatis RE, Cowen SS, Kolb DA. Innovation in professional education: steps on a journey from teaching to learning. San Francisco: Jossey Bass; 2007.
42. Boyatzis RE. Guest Edtorial: Competencies in the 21st Century. J Manag Develop. 2008;27(1):5–12.
43. Marchant R. Agenda item M14-The scope of medical regulation: physician associates. London: General Medical Council; 2015. http://www.gmcuk.org/14___The_scope_of_medical_regulation___physician_associates.pdf_64608156.pdf.
44. Boyzatis RE, Kolb DA. Assessing individuality in learning: the learning skils profile. Educ Psychol. 1991;11(3&4):279–95.
45. Boyzatis RE, Kolb DA. From learning styles to learning skills: the executive skills profile. J Manag Psychol. 1995;10(5):3–17.

Effective Hospital Leadership: Quality Performance Evaluation

7

Remigiusz Wrazen and Sherif Soliman

Hospitals have come a long way since the days of the failings of the Bristol Royal Infirmary, when the inquiry reported that there was a "*substantial excess of deaths of between 30 and 35 babies under one year old, between 1991 and 1995*" ([1], p. 241). At this time the inquiry reported that there were problems with a system of healthcare rather than with any particular individual. It was reported that the surgeons were working in silos, that there were no agreed standards and little opportunity to benchmark data. However at this time there did not appear to be any agreed standards by which to measure and assess outcomes "*… no clear national standards of care emerged against which clinicians could confidently expect to compare their performance … and so it is unlikely that any clinician would expect to do so*" ([1], p. 234).

Ten years on and a review of five of the world's leading healthcare systems, identified that senior leaders rely on performance measurement to manage relationships and to assess impact of their efforts to improve performance [2]. However, it is critical that any performance evaluation tool is not used inappropriately as "*blunt uses of measurement can undermine relationships and create perverse incentives that limit performance*" [2–4]. Performance evaluation will work well when it facilitates clinician motivation in a safe and supportive organisational culture.

This chapter will explore the importance of the development of a positive 'values based' culture in hospitals that has a focus on the development of a patient safety culture. We argue for the emphasis of performance evaluation to be centred around a positive 'patient centred/patient safety' culture to support individual professional development as well as to contribute to the wider quality improvement culture within healthcare. We argue that best practice in the individual benchmarking of consultant performance within hospitals should be promoted as part of a strategy for Continuing Quality Improvement (CQI) [5] which should not focus on outcomes only, but instead be taken further to promote discussions about organisitional change. Organisations will need to be prepared to 'disrupt' traditional ways of working (that do not add value to the patient) as hospitals pursue more innovative ways to engage patients who will become the lead focus to transform services. Globally, health care organisations have placed a strong emphasis on continuous quality improvement (CQI) as a vehicle to facilitate this change. CQI was initially pioneered by Americans W. A. Shewhart, W. Edward Deming,

R. Wrazen (✉)
Sheffield Teaching Hospitals NHS Foundation Trust, Sheffield, UK
e-mail: rwrazen@btinternet.com

S. Soliman
Faculty of Medicine, Al-Azhar Training and Development Centre, Al-Azhar University, Cairo, Egypt
e-mail: sherifsalahsoliman@gmail.com

P. Godbole et al. (eds.), *Why Hospitals Fail*, DOI 10.1007/978-3-319-56224-7_7

and Joseph Juran from the 1930s to the 1950s and later refined in Japan, with its roots in Kaizen, which emphasizes small, low-cost, low-risk improvements [6].

The word Kaizen is translated from Japanese in a number of ways, most simply as "change for the better", "Kai" means "change", "zen" means "good" [7]. A "Kaizen" is a small improvement that is made by those who do the work. It is a small, low-cost, low-risk improvement that can be easily implemented. Kaizen is an ongoing methodology and philosophy for challenging and empowering everyone in the organisation to use their creative ideas to improve their daily work. Many organizations embrace the idea of Kaizen and practice its specific principles, but they call it Continuous Improvement, Process Excellence, or Plan-Do-Study-Act instead of Kaizen [7]).

This chapter will offer a discussion of 'disruptive innovation' as a way to embrace Continuous Quality Improvement (CQI) in clinical performance evaluation. Secondly we will illustrate this with a case study to show how clinical performance evaluation can 'disrupt' our normalised thinking of performance appraisal by the use of quality improvement tools such as embedding "Kaizen", statistical process control measures and run charts. The use of QI methods within the clinical performance appraisal provides a neutral focus on performance, removing any personal or subjective focus on the individual consultant. Instead the conversation becomes a more objective discussion around improvement for the patient experience and how reflection on performance evaluation and benchmarking can provide value to the patient.

Benchmarking has been defined as "*the process of identifying and learning from good practices in other organisations*" (EFQM—European Benchmarking Code of Conduct, 2009). Clinical practice benchmarking involves structured comparison of processes and the sharing of best practices in clinical care. It is based on a quality assessment and is integrated within a CQI approach.

According to Ettorchi et al. [5] Benchmarking incorporates the following elements:

- Regularly comparing indicators (structure, activities, processes and outcomes) against best practices
- Identifying differences in outcomes through inter-organisational visits
- Seeking out new approaches in order to make improvements that will have the greatest impact on outcomes

When quality is embraced as a business strategy, organisations can develop as high performing organisations. It also gives a clear rationale for medical leaders to innovate in healthcare. Innovation in the healthcare industry has its own unique challenges. Any attempt to understand the process of innovation in healthcare must begin with an in-depth analysis of its challenges. Any attempt at modeling the process of health care innovation must take into account the health care stakeholders' unique and deliberate needs, wants and expectations [8].

Innovation can be categorised by its impact on stakeholders as nondisruptive or disruptive. Nondisruptive innovations are improving on something that already exists but in a way that allows expanded opportunities to be met, or existing problems to be solved. They may be also referred to as incremental, evolutionary, linear, or sustaining. While disruptive innovations refer to innovations that disorder old systems, create new players (for example patients leading service redesign) and create new markets (more integrated services and day case surgery) while marginalizing old ones, and deliver dramatic value to stakeholders who successfully implement and adapt to the innovation. They may be also called radical, revolutionary, transformational, or nonlinear [8].

Innovation in healthcare continues to be a driving force for health care quality. Sharing thoughts between health care staff at different levels and their leaders in a trustable and respectable environment is the main step to create new ideas. Also, involving stakeholders in the innovation process directly or indirectly will assure successful dissemination.

To support staff to work and perform their best in a new culture, with emancipatory values, fairness and ethical leadership, there is a need to have a form of quality performance evaluation. Quality as defined in Chapter 1 supports the standard IoM definition of six domains. To measure quality and performance in a particular specialty, specialty specific indicators need to be produced reflecting three different approaches: Structure, Process and Outcomes [9].

The current paradigm of medicine and surgery still gives priority to "Outcomes" over process and structure and they are still widely considered as the ultimate validators of quality of medical care, despite the fact that they do not provide insight into the strengths and weaknesses of care, and what is more likely to be of 'value' to the patient. A review of 88,069 patient complaints [10] show that the process and structure of health care is just as important as the outcomes as 15.6% of the complaints reviewed were about the treatment (outcomes) and 13.7% of complaints were about communication (structure and process) between a health care system and the patient.

7.1 A Definition of Quality for Clinical Performance Evaluation

The quality of health care has to be embedded into the process of care and continuously managed, not only controlled. Modern medicine heavily relies on guidelines and protocols derived from Evidence Based Medicine (EBM). A well-defined process based on EBM is what can be called "a medicine properly practiced". According to Donabedian quality may be defined by the structure within which processes of care happen. The assumption of this approach is that if we combine things, which we know are good for a patient (processes) with high quality facilities, equipment and staff (structure), the result of this intervention (the outcome) should be positive. However, as was outlined at the start of this chapter, without benchmarking practice against other hospitals, it is unclear if the structure, process or outcomes are optimal and in line with what is expected.

Øvretveit [11] proposes an integrated definition of quality based on a three-dimensional structure:

- Patient quality is what patients say they want.
- Professional quality is what professionals think patient needs
- Management quality is using the fewest resources, without waste, errors or delay, and within policy and legal regulations

He concludes that integrated quality development should be a balanced process in which there is no trade-off between increasing patient satisfaction, improving professional outcomes and reducing cost.

7.2 Collecting Data: Deciding on the Quality Indicators

7.2.1 Measuring for Quality Improvement

The approach [12] sets out the Department of Health's aspiration for the development and use of indicators of quality at all levels of the system, including:

- Local clinical teams using measures for benchmarking and day-to-day monitoring.

A range of quality indicators has been set but NHS organisations are also encouraged to consider developing their own local indicators.

The economic pressures in the UK put an increasing demand on NHS Tusts in terms of accountability and according to Benn et al. [13] effective monitoring of quality of service delivery is central to the capacity of an organisation or unit to maintain and improve standards of care. According to Øvretveit [14] gathering and using data are often the weakest components of improvement programmes, despite the fact that they play an essential role in monitoring and improving quality.

7.2.2 Performance Evaluation in Anaesthesia: A Case Study

Traditional methods of monitoring quality of anaesthesia relied on analysis of perioperative mortality and morbidity, not always directly related to anaesthesia (perioperative mortality less than 1% while death from anaesthesia 1 in 200,000) and anaesthetic incidents, which rely heavily on self-reporting and willingness of staff members to report them, is not a good indicator of incidence. In a systematic review of quality and safety indicators in anaesthesia, Haller et al. [15] identified 108 clinical indicators developed for anaesthesia. Many of these indicators related to surgical and ward care, and were not specific to anaesthesia. Most of the indicators identified were used as indirect measures and further steps needed to be taken to confirm a potential quality issue. The majority were based on outcomes (57%)—which poses a problem for anaesthesia, where outcomes are often not very well defined. Anaesthesia is a part of the much larger and complex treatment process and the outcome of this process obviously cannot be used to assess quality of anaesthesia alone, as indicated above. Haller et al. [15] discovered that the number of process indicators for anaesthesia was the fastest growing among all indicators. The process indicators define targets of "how things should be done" to ensure quality of anaesthesia care. Unfortunately they tend to be perceived more as "quality improvement tools" than real measures of quality and their validation is largely limited to expert opinions. Evidence that compliance with evidence-based best practice systematically results in better patient outcome [16, 17] is a significant question mark over the use of process indicators in the outcome driven healthcare.

Quality indicators of the process can be derived from nationally agreed care bundles like Surgical Site Infection (SSI), a part of High Impact Intervention program aimed at reducing the incidence and consequences of surgical site infections.

A patient undergoing surgical procedures under anaesthesia expects it to be pain free, sick free, highly personalised and a pleasant experience. Postoperative pain and postoperative nausea and vomiting (PONV) are two of the most important dimensions of quality in the postoperative period with a strong negative influence upon patient satisfaction [18]. Such data are recorded as part of recovery care plans in NHS hospitals. Ease of analysis could be improved by capturing it electronicaly but this is not commonly available in all recovery areas.

7.3 Targets and Goals

After establishing a list of quality indicators the next step would be to decide how much of a process improvement is required. Short-term targets are an essential part of Plan-Do-Study-Act cycles, while long-term goals form a part of much wider and far reaching strategies. A patient's view and expectations should be a foundation of decision-making in the process of setting goals. The choice of goals also depends on external benchmarks set by industry leaders. The Hospital can choose to achieve the same level as the "best of the best" or strive to become even better within a culture of Continuous Quality Improvement. The targets should be set in a non-arbitrary fashion by an improvement team and reflect the agreed schedule of achieving goals.

7.4 Benchmarking

In their review article Varughese et al. [19] describe benchmarking as a continuous process of measuring to identify and understand "best practices" that enable organisations to improve quality. A common misconception about benchmarking is that it means meeting a target, a numeric value based on internal or external standards set by the industry leaders. Each organisation should develop its own benchmarking to help identify the most efficient ways of working.

7.5 Run Charts and Control Charts

Run charts and control charts are the simplest graphical method that displays data plotted over time and allows for the observation of trends and patterns.

A run chart can help you spot upward and downward trends and it can show you a general picture of a process. Unfortunately run charts lack the benefit of statistical control limits. So, if they are used to adjust your process, this may add more variation to the process instead of reducing the variation.

A control chart also plots a single line of data over time, but includes upper and lower control and warning limit lines, which allow you to answer more specific questions about the process like "Is this process stable or in control?" Control limits describe the variability in the process and if any of your data are outside the limit lines, the answer is negative. You would then know that system changes may be required to make it stable.

Control charts are designed to prevent two common mistakes: (1) adjusting the process when it should be left alone; and (2) ignoring the process when it may need to be adjusted.

Statistical Process Crontrol (SPC) is a core part of a Continuous Quality Improvement (CQI) programme visioned by W. Shewart from Bell Labs in 1920s. Deming [20] built upon this work, proposing a continuous process of improvement by revising the production processes on the basis of data about processes themselves. Deming generated a list of 14 principles of management to achieve a culture of CQI (Table 7.1).

A CQI system aims to deliver the highest possible quality at the lowest possible cost and to ensure that quality becomes built into the process, not added on at the end. It allows you to see if a process is stable or not, and seeks to eliminate special cause variation for every process, leaving only random variation. When the process is not stable other tools like Ishikawa diagrams or Pareto charts can be used to identify the sources

Table 7.1 Deming [20] 14 principles of management in developing a culture of quality

1. *Create constancy of purpose* toward improvement of product and service, with the aim to become competitive and to stay in business, and to provide jobs.
2. *Adopt the new philosophy.* We are in a new economic age. Western management must awaken to the challenge, must learn their responsibilities, and take on leadership for change.
3. *Cease dependence on inspection to achieve quality.* Eliminate the need for inspection on a mass basis by building quality into the product or service in the first place.
4. *End the practice of awarding business on the basis of price tag.* Instead, minimize total cost. Move toward a single supplier for any one item, on a long-term relationship of loyalty and trust.
5. *Improve constantly and forever the system of production and service,* to improve quality and productivity, and thus constantly decrease costs.
6. *Institute on the job training.*
7. *Institute leadership.* The aim of supervision should be to help people and machines and gadgets to do a better job.
8. *Drive out fear,* so that everyone may work effectively for the company.
9. *Break down barriers between departments.* People in research, design, sales, and production must work as a team, to foresee problems of production and in use that may be encountered with the product or service.
10. *Eliminate slogans, exhortations, and targets* for the work force asking for zero defects and new levels of productivity. Such exhortations only create adversarial relationships, as the bulk of the causes of low quality and low productivity belong to the system and thus lie beyond the power of the work force.
11. *Remove barriers that rob the hourly worker of his right to pride of workmanship.* The responsibility of supervisors must be changed from sheer numbers to quality.
12. *Remove barriers that rob people in management and in engineering of their right to pride of workmanship.* This means, inter alia, abolishment of the annual or merit rating and of management by objective.
13. *Institute a vigorous program of education and self-improvement.*
14. *The transformation is everybody's job.* Put everybody in the company to work to accomplish the transformation.

of the excessive variation. If the special cause variation makes quality worse it should be eliminated, whereas if it improves quality it should be embedded in the process.

An improvement team makes all the decisions about what if anything needs to be improved and the steps to take after analyzing results from the charts. Understanding variation and having knowledge about special cause variation allows the devising of a process improvement plan and implementing PDSA cycles. This includes designing/re-designing the process, implementing change according to the design, studying results and finally revising practice to adopt or abandon change.

In no other field can the rewards of this effort be greater than in healthcare, where improved quality not only improves the quality of service but it can actually improve the quality of a patient's life.

7.6 Data Analysis

ORMIS is a live clinical management perioperative data-collection system, which the Hospital procured in 2004 and has been implemented across all the main theatres, recovery units and theatre Admission Units. It has allowed the Hospital to view the peri-operative pathway in great detail observing activity and utilisation of resources at individual consultant and patient level along with costs per minute. It collects a full record of events throughout the process. It is able to provide all stakeholders with robust information relating to their practices and outcomes. ORMIS has provided information, which has helped the Hospital to increase the quality of services which has delivered efficiencies and savings in excess of 50 million pounds. Data from ORMIS has been used in aiding the establishment of NICE guidelines about perioperative warming [21] and in support of efficiency projects such as "Productive Operating Theatre".

In addition to this in the Post Anaesthetic Care Unit, wireless tablets are used to record the Recovery Care Plan and manual electronic charting. Data collected include vital signs like temperature, blood pressure, heart rate, oxygen blood saturation, respiratory rate as well as values for pain, sedation and nausea scores. There is one device per bed space, mounted on a mobile cart and transmitting data wirelessly to the server. Users input data with a stylus and find it quicker than charting on paper. Other recovery areas collect all this data on paper charts included in the patients notes.

Temperature upon arrival in recovery and time spent in recovery are important aspects of a patient's experience [13]. Collecting data about pain and nausea will give a more complete picture of perioperative anaesthetic care but analysing recovery times should be a good approximation of the same. A patient suffering postoperative nausea and vomiting or suffering excessive postoperative pain or sedation require specific interventions, which will delay meeting discharge criteria. The need to warm the patient to the desired temperature in recovery can result in prolonged stay. Recovery time is an indirect indicator and allows triggering a peer review of specific cases to assess a quality of immediate perioperative anaesthetic care of an individual patient. An increase in recovery time may result in a logjam of patients leaving the operating room leading to further delays or cancelations.

Throughout the recovery areas of the hospital, data are stored in ORMIS for timing points of arrival, meeting discharge criteria and departure. For the purposes of this case study, data sets were obtained with recovery times recorded for patients who underwent a laparoscopic cholecystectomy in the period of thirteen months between July 1st 2011 and August 1st 2012.

All patients undergoing laparoscopic cholecystectomy received a general anaesthetic with endotracheal intubation. Differences in anaesthetic agents used should not be great, nausea and vomiting is common and therefore appropriate prophylaxis should be administered. Pain levels are predictable and pain should be treated accordingly. From an anaesthesia point of view this is a fairly uniform procedure and the expectation is that outcomes should be similar.

7.7 Data Analysis Related to Laparoscopic Cholecystectomy Recovery

Between July 2011 and August 2012 487 patients had a cholecystectomy performed by 15 surgeons and 67 anaesthetists. This group of anaesthetists can be divided onto 37 consultants and 30 trainees.

Average recovery time for the whole data set is 74 min. The range is between 0 min and 487 min. Figure 7.1 indicates average recovery times for individual anaesthetists.

There are also eight patients without recorded name of the anaesthetist. These patients have been included in analysis (Fig. 7.2) of calculating overall mean and mean recovery times for individual surgeons (Fig. 7.3).

Corrected value of average recovery time is 78 min. Average recovery time in a consultant group is 85 min comparing with 70 min for trainees group. One explanation could be the fact that consultants have to anaesthetise more high-risk cases. Further analysis using for example ASA scoring which correlates well with perioperative risk could help to establish more comparable groups of patients. Dividing the trainee group into senior (post FRCA examination) and more junior one could also provide a more complete picture. Recording of ASA scoring is available in ORMIS, but for the majority of patients it relies on voluntary input by an anaesthetist or a surgeon. In our data set ASA was recorded for 124 patients out of 458 patients included in this analysis.

In this example these bar charts indicating general trends tell very little about individual performance and can be very misleading. It is important to be cautious in using such data in a simplistic way in performance evaluation.

Another chart (Fig. 7.3) demonstrates that average recovery time might also to some degree depend on a surgeon performing an operation. In practice senior registrars very often perform surgery, which is recorded under a consultant name and these data would require further analysis to establish a convincing link between recovery time and operating surgeon.

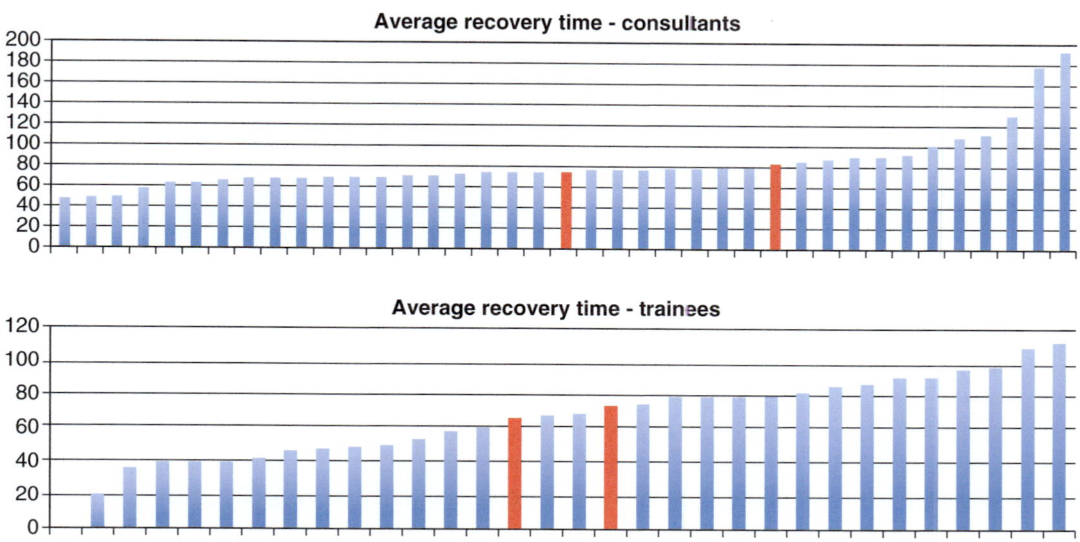

Fig. 7.1 Detailed analysis of data revealed that there were 25 patients in the data set with recovery times of 0 min and further four patients with recovery times below 8 min. These patients have most probably gone to critical care bypassing recovery and for purpose of this example they have been removed from the data set to make it more representative

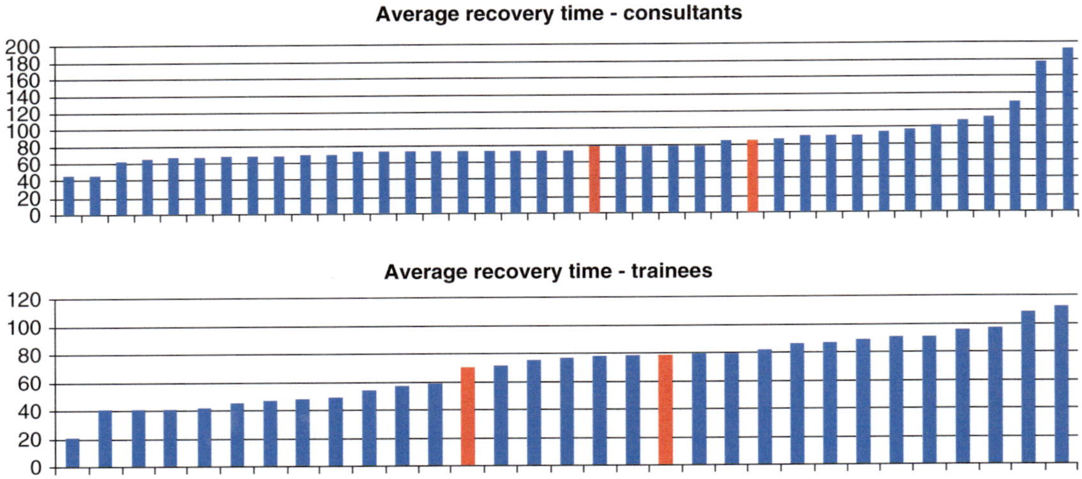

Fig. 7.2 For example a consultant anaesthetist with the shortest average time only anaesthetised two cases and a consultant anaesthetist with the longest average time only anesthetised one case. The consultant with second longest average time anaesthetised four cases in total, including the patient with the longest recorded recovery time (487 min). Other patient's recovery times for this individual were below the consultant average

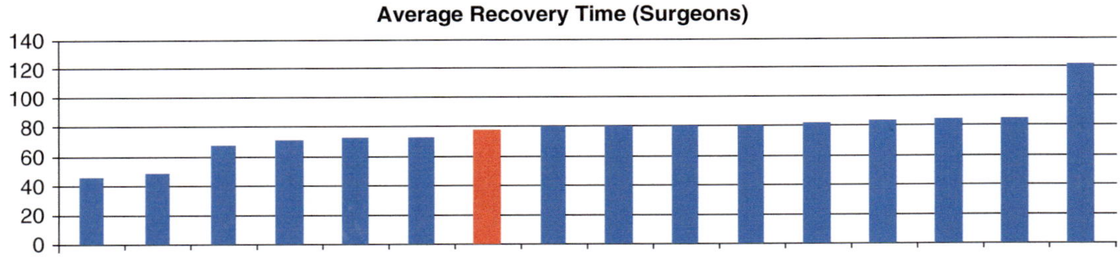

Fig. 7.3 These data are only useful in so much as they can be used as indirect indicators or trend indicators. There are numerous factors influencing a length of recovery stay and one has to consider all those factors before reaching final conclusions about the quality of process and the performance of the individual. To try and assess individual doctor performance one has to look much more closely and try to establish at first if individual performance is an established and controlled process

This can be looked at using the run chart and the control chart. In Fig. 7.4 there are examples of such charts showing some considerable variations. Without review of other data like nausea, sedation and pain scores it is difficult to explain such a variation. It can be also associated with a surgeon, with whom this consultant anaesthetist works during controlled periods. Some other perioperative factors like specific interventions in the process or changes of structure within which process occur might be responsible for periodic increases in recovery times.

Figure 7.5 shows different examples of control charts derived from our data. Chart (a) shows a lot of variability. At this stage it is difficult to tell reasons behind such a large differences. A review of consultant practice can give some more information as to which other factors have to be considered. Chart (b) is an example of a much more controlled process with some special cause variation. Analysis of cases with longer recovery times can give an answer to the question about what went wrong and why such extended time was given to a patient.

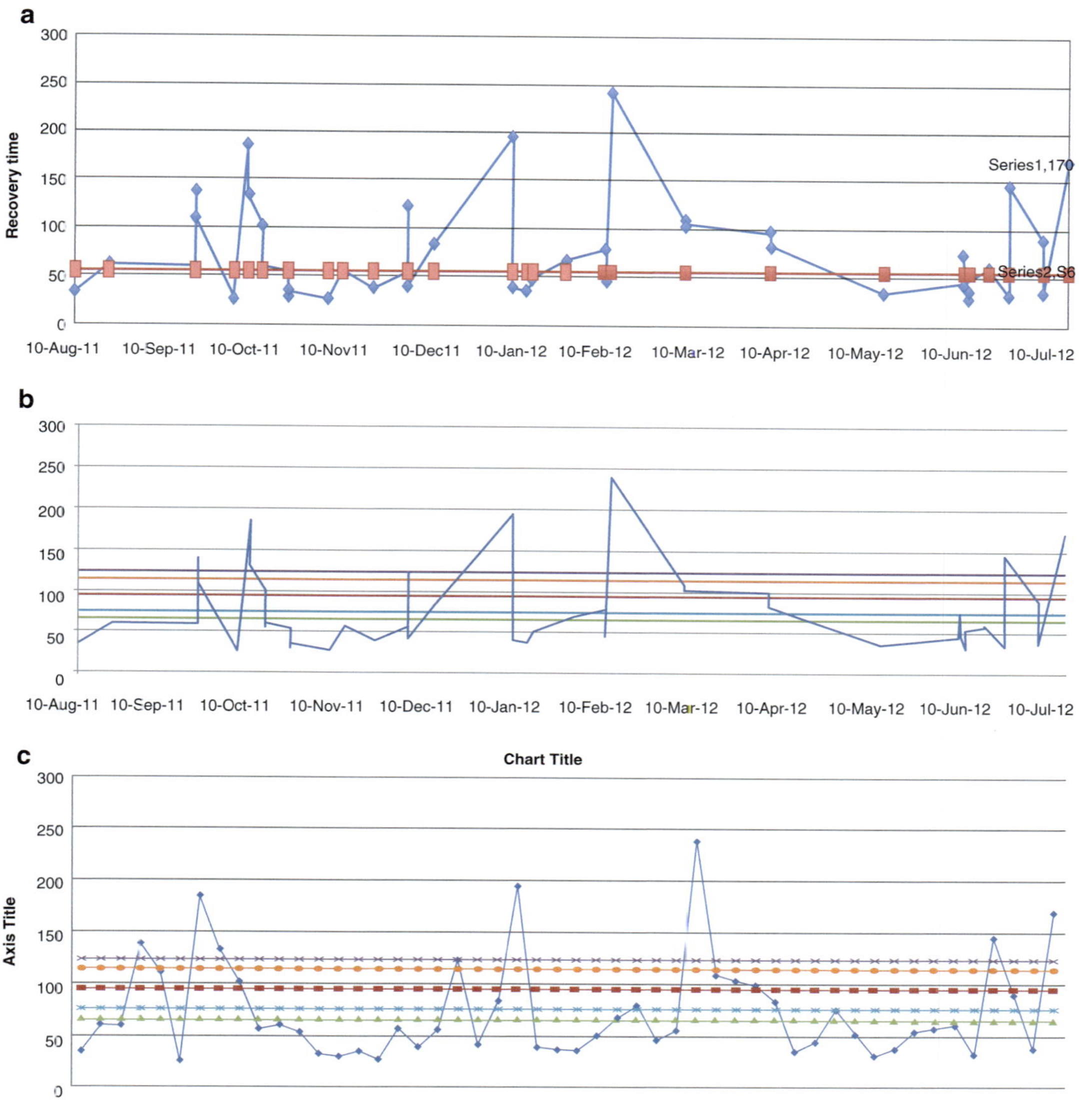

Fig. 7.4 (**a**) Run chart of recovery times for consultant X. The *red line* indicates median value. (**b**) Control chart of recovery times for consultant X. The *red line* marks the mean. The *purple line* marks upper control limit (+3SD) and the *orange line* marks upper warning limit (+2SD). The *blue line* marks lower warning limit (−2SD) and the *green line* marks lower control limit (−3SD). (**c**) Control chart of recovery times for consultant X. This time events are spread evenly over time

In some situations when a target has been set it is more appropriate to use p-chart. In this example we can decide to establish the maximum recovery time after laparoscopic cholecystectomy. The p-charts using the percentage of patients fulfilling the set criteria for our data will look like in Fig. 7.6. The blue dots indicate a percentage of patients with recovery times meeting the target time or below the target each month. This process is in control because the plotted line stays within control limits.

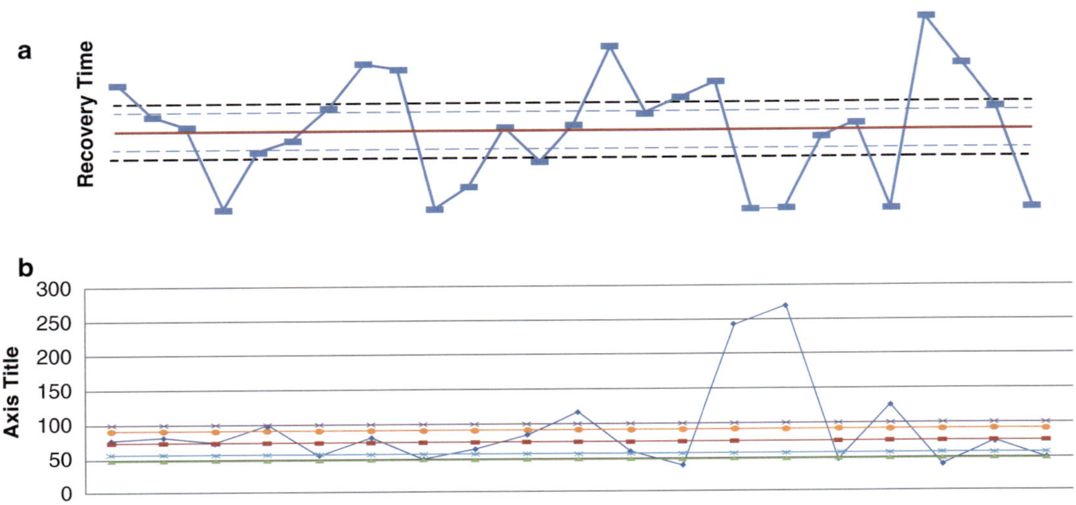

Fig. 7.5 Control chart for consultant anaesthetist (**a**) shows significant variations and uncontrolled process. Control chart for consultant anaesthetist (**b**) shows a period of controlled process followed by significant disruption (special cause variation)

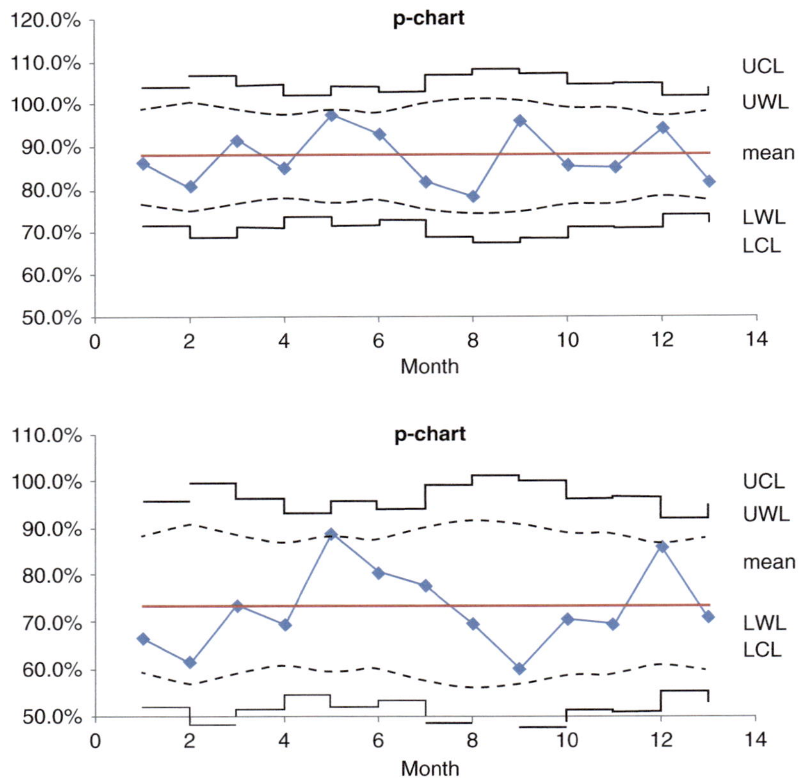

Fig. 7.6 P-charts—*top* to *bottom* is 120, 90, 60 and 45 min target to meet discharge criteria

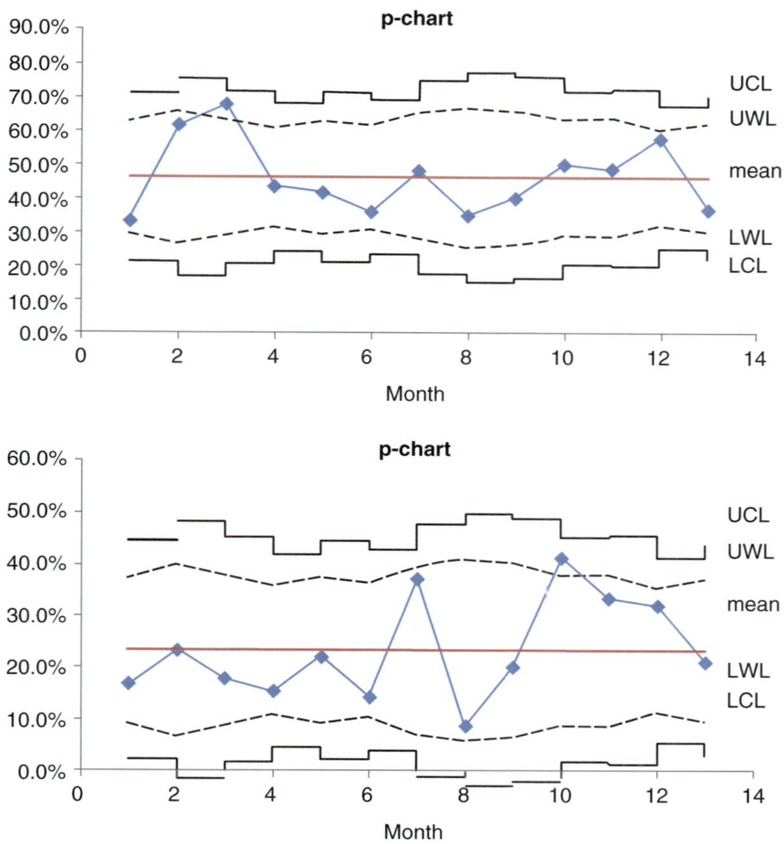

Fig. 7.6 (continued)

7.8 Limitations and Reliability of Data Collection System

ORMIS is a well-established system at the hospital and is used to collect a wide range of data. Staff are familiar with it and are accustomed to inputting the data, but unfortunately some data required for continous improvement and performance evaluation are not mandatory and rely on either an anaesthetist or a surgeon's willingness to report. ASA score is one example of such data that can be very useful. Only two recovery areas are equipped with electronic means of capturing recovery data while others collect this data on paper, which makes it impossible to gather and analyse data in a continuous way. It has not been possible to extend this service to the other areas due to the capital and maintenance costs involved.

Recovery adheres to strict discharge protocols based on guidelines set by national professional bodies and an agreed local set of recommendation. This allows eliminating possible variation and bias from decision-making process. The discharge process is supported by a set of recorded parameters, which as discussed earlier can form part of quality improvement system. These parameters are recorded using standarised and reliable methods.

7.9 How Well Is the Department Doing?

The answer to this question depends on the question: how well we would like to be doing?

The anaesthetic department at the hospital does not currently purposefully collect quality indicator data. Data that can be potentially be used to support the quality improvement process is captured routinely as part of the perioperative pathway and recovery care plan, but the majority are recorded on paper, making it impossible to perform statistical process control.

Data analysis in the example for this chapter showed some significant variations between individual's performances and for single individual, for what should be fairly uniformed practice. On the other hand the analysis of data with a range of target discharge times showed a controlled process. It is argued that there is room for improvement in terms of consistency of individual performance and that it would be useful to use these data to benchmark against other hospitals across the country. Internal benchmarking in this instance can be useful in identifying the best practice, which can be shared and ingrained in the process. Once the process is stable a more ambitious target can be set such as 30 min discharge time (in line with the clinical protocol) for laparoscopic cholecystectomy. This can significantly offload recovery and help avoid the previously mentioned potential logjam.

Once the process is stable and a new standard of care established a continuous process of managing quality should collect quality data and feed back to the department to encourage engagement with the process [22].

Recent research [23] looked at using such data with a national government funded study, and concluded that it was important to identify the way in which feedback is given to doctors. The success of the quality improvement process depends upon providing feedback on performance in a more objective and scientific way, with a clear rationale to drive system improvement. This promotes a 'no blame' culture and instead encourages a team-work approach to improving and standardising quality care for patients. The researchers [23] found that implementation of basic feedback had no effect on quality of anaesthetic service, but the implementation of enhanced feedback resulted in significant improvement in quality indicators. The study showed that clinicians value and respond extremely positively to interventions combining data with user in the context of a specific procedure, as well as having a "willingness to interact with a sustained and comprehensive feedback protocol to understand variations in care". Researchers concluded that "The results support the potential of quality monitoring and feedback interventions as quality improvement mechanisms and provide insight into the positive response of clinicians to this type of initiative, including documentation of the experiences of anaesthetists that participated as users and co-designers of the feedback".

References

1. Kennedy I. The report of the public inquiry into children's heart surgery at the Bristol Royal Infirmary 1984–1995 – Learning from Bristol Department of Health, UK; 2001.
2. Baker GR. The roles of leaders in high performing health care systems. London: The Kings Fund; 2011. www.kingsfund.org.uk.
3. Freeman T. Using performance indicators to improve health care quality in the public sector: a review of the literature. Health Serv Manage Res. 2002;15(2):12–37.
4. Marshall MN, Davies HTO. Performance measurement and management of healthcare professionals – some topical issues. Dis Manag Health Out. 2000;7(6):305–14.
5. Ettorchi-Tardy A, Levif M, Michel P. Benchmarking: a method for calculating quality improvement in health. Healthcare Policy. 2012;7(4):e101–19.
6. Jacobson GH, Streiff N, McCoin R, Lescallette SR, Slovis CM. Kaizen: a method of process improvement in the emergency department. Acad Emerg Med. 2009;16(12):1341–9. Accessed on line at http://onlinelibrary.wiley.com/doi/10.1111/j.1553-2712.2009.00580.x/full.
7. Graban M, Swartz JE. Health care Kaizen. Engaging front-line staff in sustainable continuous improvements. Accessed online at https://books.google.com.sa/books?isbn=1439872961. 2012.
8. Omachonu VK, Einspruch NG. Innovation in healthcare delivery systems: a conceptual framework.

Public Sec Innov J. 2010;15(1.) Article 2. Accessed online at http://www.innovation.cc/scholarly-style/omachonu_healthcare_3innovate2.pdf.
9. Donabedian A. Evaluating the quality of medical care. Milbank Q. 2005;83(4):691–729.
10. Reader TW, Gillespie A, Roberts J. Patient complaints in helthcare systems: a systematic review and coding taxonomy (May 29) BMJ Quality and Safety. 2014.
11. Øvretveit J. Health service quality. Oxford: Blackwell Scientific Press; 1992.
12. Information Centre. Measuring for quality improvement: the approach accessed online at http://www.dh.gov.uk/en/Publicationsandstatistics/Letters|andcirculars/Dearcolleagueletters/DH_090444. 2009.
13. Benn J, Arnold G, Wei I, Riley C, Aleva F. Using quality indicators in anaesthesia: feeding back data to improve care. Br J Anaesth. 2012;109(1):80–91.
14. Øvretveit J. The Norwegian approach to integrated quality development. J Manag Med. 2001;15(2):125–41.
15. Haller G, Stoelwinder J, Myles PS, McNeil J. Quality and safety indicators in anesthesia: a systematic review. Anesthesiology. 2009;110:1158–75.
16. Bahtsevani C, Uden G, Willman A. Outcomes of evidence-based clinical practice guidelines: a systematic review. Int J Technol Assess Health Care. 2004;20:427–33.
17. Grimshaw JM, Russell IT. Effect of clinical guidelines on medical practice: a systematic review of rigorous evaluations. Lancet. 1993;342:1317–22.
18. Macario A. Which clinical anesthesia outcomes are important to avoid? The perspective of patients. Anesth Analg. 1999;89:652.
19. Varughese, et al. Quality of pediatric anesthesia. Pediatr Anesth. 2010;20:684–96.
20. Deming WE. Out of the crisis. MIT Press; 1986.
21. NICE. CG65 Perioperative hypothermia (inadvertent). Accessed online at: http://guidance.nice.org.uk/CG65/NICEGuidance/pdf/English. 2008.
22. De Vos M, Graafmans W, Kooistra M, Meijboom B, Van Der Voort P, Westert G. Using quality indicators to improve hospital care: a review of the literature. Int J Qual Health Care. 2009;21:119–29.
23. Benn J, Arnold G, D'Lima D, Wei I, Moore J, Aleva F. Evaluation of a continuous monitoring and feedback initiative to improve quality of anaesthetic care: a mixed-methods quasi-experimental study. Health Serv Deliv Res. 2015;3(32.) National Institute for Health Research.

8 What Is a Team and Effective Team Working

David Johnson

From the times of our ancestors, the need to succeed has been paramount to our survival, and it should not be much of a surprise to note the more effective the team, the more likely the chances were of surviving. ([1], p. 5)

8.1 Introduction

The introductory quote from Crother-Laurin seems to have become embedded in the culture of organisations across the world. Indeed organisations large, small or somewhere in between spend huge sums of money every year on team building, relationship building and building trust. Senior leader development programmes tend to focus on these issues, (although they might not actually call them team work). It would seem, when unpicked and however it is described, these concepts are at the heart of successful leadership and successful organisations across many sectors.

The instinctive answer to the question of 'how can we get the most out of the people who work here?' when a problem arises is "we will get a team onto it".

D. Johnson
Department of Social Work Social Care and Community Studies, Sheffield Hallam University, Sheffield, UK
e-mail: David.Johnson@shu.ac.uk

As is often the case, although 'teams' seem to be a simple concept, the reality of creating a successful team is far more complex. Teams are often talked about in the context of sports and sometimes useful analogies to organisational life can be made. The UK has an elite professional soccer/football league called the Premier League. Vast sums of money are expended in buying and paying the wages of the best players that are sourced from across the world. In 2016 a team called Leicester City won the Premier League. At the start of the season they were predicted to be relegated from the league. Leicester's entire squad of players cost less than the price of buying one player that was transferred into a rival team, their squad of players cost eight times less than a team that came fourth in the league; yet they still won. Often press reporters would comment on team spirit and team identify, they would talk about how the team worked for each other, these aspects were described as the critical factors in their success. There are many factors in this story that do resonate with what we know about health care teams, and it would seem that just having the best people doesn't always produce the best result.

There are, it would seem, many who seek alchemic texts on the subject of team working, many that look for an elixir that will provide them with their perfect team. If only this was possible, and the recipe for such a potion (or poison) could be written down in a chapter like

P. Godbole et al. (eds.), *Why Hospitals Fail*, DOI 10.1007/978-3-319-56224-7_8

this and once formulated distributed to the staff group. This chapter doesn't seek to promise to deliver such a magical potion, it will identify pitfalls and offer suggestions to help develop your effective team, but, as a word of caution, as with many things worth doing, this is hard ongoing, often unrecognised and unrewarded work. The team is almost a living thing, an entity that needs nurturing and caring for if it is to grow, succeed and achieve all that it could achieve. As with a plant you might get away with sticking a seed in a plant pot with some soil and putting it somewhere in the garden and it might produce the odd flower; but the gardener knows that with care, through pruning, feeding, sunshine and water it will truly flourish and be bountiful in delivering whatever it is designed to do (and it often gives so much more) and so it is with teams.

Many leaders in many sectors including the health sector attempt to foster a culture that encourages teamwork but they often tend to view teams as an approach to getting the business done. There is often very little thinking or questioning about if deploying this team at this time is actually the best approach to getting this aspect of our business done. Equally there is often little thought given to how the team will form, how a group of individuals will initially interact to reap the benefit of the team, how the team will deal with its own ongoing development and identify. There is only the belief that the team will perform and therefore deliver. Crother-Laurin [1] takes a slightly different view she believes that effective teams should not be a goal of the organisation but they will emerge as a result of healthy leadership.

Before we dive headlong into the deep end of team working I wonder if it is worth exploring the shallows and considering the viability of a number of different working options.

8.2 Simple Starting Point

The first question to be considered is why bother at all, is there actually a need to work together? It is often said that as a simple starting point if a person can achieve their goals without involving others they will. The foundations stones of most organisations and teams are laid, however, when it is no longer possible for goals to be achieved by working on your own, only by joining with others will common goals be reached. Therefore, this time of joining, of becoming a team or a group is fundamental to the way that resources, power and tasks are divided up within an organisation.

8.3 Teams or Groups

It is difficult to imagine how anyone, working within today's complex, integrated health and social care settings, no matter how brilliant, could achieve the best outcomes for a patient by always working alone. The next question therefore is do they work in a team or in a group. Indeed there is a lot of discrepancy within literature with regard to this question. Mullins [2] even suggest that the terms are often interchanged with little rationale or thought for the use of one term instead of the other, he believes it isn't easy to differentiate clearly between a group and a team.

Mullins [2] does, however, identify some criteria that will, he feels, if met lead to the formation of a group identify instead of a team identity.

Looking across a range of definitions (including Mullins) a group could be defined as,

A collection of people who share most, if not all of the following characteristics:

- There is a clear definable membership
- The group perceives themselves as a group, there is a group consciousness
- There is a sense of shared purpose amongst members

But

- Each member has the ability to act in a unitary manner,
- Fundamentally there is no need for a collective increase in performance as a result their activity
- and they are not mutually accountable

Again team definitions are many and varied across the literature, however, when looking for a common definition for teams Northouse [3] offers that team members are interdependent, they have a common goal and must co-ordinate their activities if they are to achieve their goal. Crainer ([4], p. 287) states "When a number of people have a common goal and recognise that personal success is dependent upon the success of others, they are all interdependent".

The difference then between what is described as a group and what is a team would be that yes, group members will work together on issues and there will be perhaps a sense of a common direction, (but not a common goal). Fundamentally members of a group do not have to rely on the work of others in order to achieve their personal goals, they are not interdependent. By working together in a group there is no real need or desire for a collective increase in performance. Within a team an individual can only succeed if the team succeed.

Katzenbach and Smith (1993) described five different models of group/team working. Although written many years ago, it does continue to have a relevance to this subject and is worth exploring further.

8.3.1 Working Group

A working group is collection of people who work together, primarily to share information, best practice or perspectives and to make decisions that help each individual perform within their area of responsibility. There is no realistic or truly desired common purpose; no increase in performance as a consequence of working together and of course, there is no mutual accountability for each other's actions and therefore no collective increase in performance as a result of interactions. As a member of a working group, I hope that all my colleagues within the group benefit from our interaction with each other, but fundamentally I need the group to give me what I need, in order to do well for myself. Working groups are endemic in most organisations and a lot is achieved through them but they are not teams and as Katzenbach and Smith (2006, p. xviii) state "the untapped potential of teams in organisations is enormous." It would seem that in the austerity driven world that dominate the public sector and in particular the health care sector we, more than ever, need to understand teams.

8.3.2 Pseudo Team

This is a group for which there could be significant increase in performance by working together and there is even an opportunity to do this. But the people within the group are just not focussed on collective performance and they are not really trying to achieve together. The people associated with this group will probably call themselves and be called a team by others, but they don't work in ways that develop mutual accountability, they don't their shape goals together, they don't develop the benefits of team working, they don't perhaps even have complementary skills, they are a Pseudo team. Katzenbach and Smith [5] describe a pseudo team as the weakest of all groups, when considering issues of performance. This group is perhaps the biggest lost opportunity.

8.3.3 Potential Team

This is a team where the situation does suggest there could be a significant need for an increase in performance as a consequence of their combined interaction. The team is really is trying to improve performance by working together. This team is working towards mutual accountability but it hasn't actually achieved it yet. There is often a need for a greater understanding of what can be achieved together, common goals are fuzzy and not well developed and more time is needed to work out common approaches to working. This is a team that, as the name suggests, with a little more nurturing could really see big increases in performance as a consequence of its effective interaction, only, it has quite managed this at the moment, but it is travelling in the right direction and is worth developing further.

8.3.4 Real Team

Katzenbach and Smiths [5] describe a real team as a small number of people (usually less than 10) who have complementary skill, who are committed to a common purpose and common goals and have an approach to work that they all agree upon. Of significant importance to this team is that team members agree that they hold themselves mutually accountable for the team's performance.

8.3.5 High Performance Teams

Their final category was defined as a high performance team. This definition included all of the characteristics of a real team but added that team members are "deeply committed" to one another's personal growth and success. They conclude that high performing teams are very rare creatures that need nurturing and, if you have experienced working within one you are both lucky and will have understood the advantages of working in this way. In empirical discussion with colleagues, if this definition found a resonance with someone, there is always a contemplative and reflective smile about how good these times had been, about how much had been achieved and about how significant this period had been in their professional development. There is always an enormous amount of goodwill extended towards the others members of this team.

An exercise that asks participants to analyse all of the teams and groups that they are a part of and then categorise them into the groupings that Katzenbach and Smith [5] describe often produces interesting reflections. It might be a good idea to do this exercise now, to think about all the different aspects that are a part of the groups and teams that you are in and identify how they would map against these definitions.

So does it matter how you would describe the working arrangement you have with colleagues? Usually after compiling the list in the exercise above, a number of different (perhaps less than satisfactory) arrangements are identified yet organisations still on the whole seem to survive and even thrive.

The National Health Service in the United Kingdom is a very large employer, indeed it is one of the biggest employers in the world. In 2012 it employed about 1.4 million people, and was classified as the biggest employer in Britain and the fifth biggest employer in the world. Each year this organisation carries out a survey of its staff to determine their satisfaction with their employer. Amongst other things, the survey asks if participants work in a team, in about 90% of cases the answer that is returned is yes. So 90% of NHS employees believe that they work in a team. They are then asked further questions regarding clear objectives, reviewing common goals and working together, all factors believed to be significantly important in teams. West [6] considered their responses and identified that actually only 40% of people worked in real teams, and that 50% of respondent worked in pseudo teams. Clearly a huge misperception of how teams work by a lot of NHS employees. But the really interesting and important part of West's [6] research concluded, after analysis of data, that the higher the percentage of people working in pseudo teams the higher the incidents of bullying and harassment of staff from a range of groups, the higher the levels of injuries to staff at work, the higher the level of assaults on staff by patient groups and most significantly the higher the level of witnessed errors that could harm a patient. As would be expected the data revealed the opposite in people that worked in real teams with fewer injuries, errors, assault and harassment. Real team workers would also miss work far less often; there is less absenteeism within real teams. From an organisational perspective, based on the NHS staff survey, real teams deliver so much more on so many levels.

As a final and perhaps most important point, West [6] even identifies lower levels of patient mortality associated with real team working. He believes that as little as 5% more staff working in real teams would deliver a decrease in mortality of 3.3% or in more simple terms around 40 people per year per hospital would not die. This is an incredible claim; at the beginning of this chapter Crother-Laurin [1] described how throughout history, people that work in teams stood a greater chance of survival than those that didn't. According to West's research it would seem that the reality of this quote for a patient that is being worked on/with by a health team is stark!

West [6] believes that there are in effect two functions to team working. The first he calls "task functioning" the second he calls the "social emotional climate". Charles Handy [7] described a similar concept; he identified the two purposes as an organisational purpose and an individual purpose.

Organisational purpose	Individual purpose
Distribution of work	Satisfy social or affiliation needs
Management and control of work	Establish a concept of self
Problem solving and decision making	Gain help and support to carry out objectives
Information and idea collection	Share and help in common activity or purpose
Information processing	
Testing and ratifying decisions	
Co-ordination and liaison	
Increasing commitment and involvement	
Negotiation and conflict resolution	

West believed that reflecting upon all of these areas, alongside reflecting on common goals and common ways of working are essential if teams are to function. Often there is quite rightly a focus on the organisational purpose of team, but if the individual purpose of being part team is not addressed, as time progresses, we don't have a team!

8.4 The Team Meeting

At the start of the chapter we talked about how the team is almost a living thing and that it needed nurturing. In many health care settings "team meetings" are considered a way of getting business done. It is true they are an excellent vehicle for passing information on, but do they really achieve all that they could achieve? Chronic busyness is endemic in organisations and is often worn as a "badge of honour". Colleagues compete to convince each other of who has the busiest life ([8], p. 4). As a consequence the opportunity to spend time reflecting on the team (and not the task) is sometimes considered a luxury that we just haven't got time for. Managers will often want to pass on performance and task information but, reflecting on the nature of the team, how it functions, what are its common goals and common ways of doing things, well, its all a bit abstract, a bit unnecessary, a bit uncomfortable and of course fraught with danger of personal disagreement and conflict, perhaps best to avoid then and get on with the job.

Of course I just don't agree; it is perhaps at busy and difficult times that this "unnecessary navel gazing" is actually most needed where the benefits and support of effective team working can be best realised. It is at these times that we need the team to function at its best, and it can only do this if it is able to take the time to consider and embrace all the aspect that make up a team not just the task and performance bits. Bridges [9] when discussing how to lead change described how sometime leaders are focussed on technical competency, (e.g. the best surgical procedure for the speciality), but they do not see working with people as necessarily their strongest suite and therefore they will avoid it if at all possible, Bridges acknowledges that working with people is not at all easy, it is however essential and cannot be avoided. West [6] described creating team environments where people feel positive and that if this can be achieved, team members will be far more willing to go the extra mile for each other. He felt that the idea that we can create effective teams by focussing on performance only and ignoring the emotional needs of team members is simply a false premise.

Finally a word of warning, Teams may have thin skin.

As stated throughout it is my belief that the team is almost a living entity, the benefits of team working have been stated many times, the work that is required to nurture the team also have been stated. Writing in 1983 about a team of social workers who worked in a hospital Nason ([10], p. 43) reflected on the vulnerability of effective teams. He felt there are that many more forces that can potentially pull teams apart compared to the forces that can hold a team together.

The forces that hold them together as "patient need, institutional support, respect and friendship".

Whilst the forces that tear teams apart include "contradictory institutional priorities, professional rivalries, misunderstanding the role of the patient, personal competitiveness and a lack of understanding of the collaborative problem solving process".

He described this as the team having thin skin, although written a long time ago I still come across many health care teams that have incredibly thin skins, does yours?

References

1. Crother-Laurin C. Effective teams a symptom of effective leadership. J Qual Particip. 2006;29(3).
2. Mullins LJ. Management and organisational behaviour. 10th ed. Upper Saddle River: Prentice Hall; 2013.
3. Northouse PG. Leadership theory and practice. 6th ed. Thousand Oaks: Sage; 2013.
4. Crainer S. Key management ideas: thinkers that changed the management world. 3rd ed. Upper Saddle River: Prentice Hall; 1998.
5. Katzenbach JR, Smith DK. The wisdom of teams; creating the high performance organisation. Boston: Harvard Business School Press; 1993.
6. West MA. Effective teamwork practical lessons from organisational research. 3rd ed. Hoboken: Wiley-Blackwell; 2012.
7. Handy C. Understanding organisation. 4th ed. London: Penguin Books; 1993.
8. Neault R. Sustainability: a new look at healthy people and workplaces. Revista Española de Orientación y Psicopedagogia. 2009;20(1):3–8.
9. Bridges W. Managing transition, making the most of change. London: Nicholas Brealey Publishing Limited; 1995.
10. Nason F. Diagnosing the hospital team. Soc Work Health Care. 1983;9(2):25–45.

9 Effective Team Working in Hospitals

Jeff Perring

9.1 Introduction

Jane was 8 months old when she was brought to the Emergency Department (ED) by her parents. She had been unwell overnight and that morning her mother noticed some spots on her chest and arms. Jane was seen by the triage nurse who immediately called over one of the department doctors to examine her. It looked like Jane had sepsis, an infection of her blood, and needed treatment immediately. The ED consultant was called as were the pediatric registrar and nurse.

It soon became clear that Jane was extremely unwell and needed help with her breathing, her blood pressure and her blood clotting. The doctors needed to take over Jane's breathing for her, a procedure usually undertaken by anesthetists. The anesthetic registrar was called, who immediately contacted her consultant because of the seriousness of the situation.

During this time the pediatric registrar, following discussion with his consultant, was calling the regional pediatric retrieval team recognizing that Jane would need to be treated in a regional pediatric intensive care unit (PICU), situated in a hospital 30 miles away. Following this call the retrieval team was mobilized whilst the intensive care consultant gave on-going advice on Jane's treatment until the retrieval team arrived.

On arrival the retrieval and local teams worked together for a number of hours to stabilize Jane before she was transferred to the PICU. Following her transfer, Jane was handed over to the PICU team who continued to care for her over the next 5 days as she slowly improved. When Jane no longer required intensive care she was transferred to the ward under the pediatric team before being discharged home to continue her recovery.

This is one example of the work taking place in hospitals across the globe and illustrates the number of teams that a single patient may come into contact with during their stay in hospital. The teams specialize in particular areas of care and together provide the knowledge and expertise needed to care for the patient as a whole. The teams in this example included the retrieval team, the PICU team and the pediatric ward team. However, there is one team that was different, the resuscitation team that developed during Jane's care in the ED. This team was more ad hoc and began with members of the ED staff, then included pediatric and anesthetic staff before finally working with the retrieval team.

Over recent years the patient safety agenda has put more emphasis on clinical teams and their effective working. In particular this relates to the patient safety agenda where a 5% increase in team performance has been estimated to potentially save 5000 lives annually in the United States [1] based upon an annual death rate due to

J. Perring
Sheffield Children's NHS Foundation Trust,
Sheffield, UK
e-mail: Jeff.Perring@sch.nhs.uk

P. Godbole et al. (eds.), *Why Hospitals Fail*, DOI 10.1007/978-3-319-56224-7_9

medical error of 98,000 [2] which was more recently estimated to be 251,454 [3].

This chapter will look at hospital teams, their structure and function and how these can influence their effectiveness. We will then consider how team training and other interventions can be used to positively influence this effectiveness. Finally, we will consider in more detail the ad hoc or 'fluid team' that developed in the ED because in in healthcare, these teams come together infrequently, when patient's are at their sickest and therefore most in need of good, effective, teamwork.

9.2 Teams

Teams have been described as two or more individuals, with the required knowledge and skills to undertake roles and tasks to achieve a common goal or goals [4]. For a team to be effective it must achieve these goals efficiently and to an acceptable standard. To do this, teams need to be able to complete the processes required (taskwork) but must also work together to support these processes. This teamwork includes situational awareness, mutual support and leadership alongside the ability to communicate both internally, between team members and externally, with other teams in a structured manner [5].

However, the process is more complicated than this in that there is a network of interactions between individuals within the team (Fig. 9.1), some of which will be task orientated whilst others will be directed more towards the team [6]. For example, whilst Jane was in the ED some team members would have been treating her through the giving intravenous fluids and antibiotics, whilst others would have been undertaking more team related actions such as talking with Jane's parents to find a possible cause for her illness and asking advice from of the intensive care consultant. Leadership would have been required to coordinate these actions but this needed to take place whilst the hierarchy or power gradients within the team were levelled to ensure that the team worked as an internal network to provide the mutual support required to reduce the risk of poor performance [7].

These aspects of teamwork are now more commonly described as human factors, which describes the behaviour of individuals and their interaction 'with each other and with their environment' [8].

Hospitals are made up of many and various teams that interact with each other and the organisation (Table 9.1). For clinical teams the most important of these interactions is the horizontal one with other clinical teams to enable continuing care of a patient. This is highlighted in Jane's story but may even be seen when considering a child with simple appendicitis who will move through a number of teams as their care progresses, from the Emergency Department to the ward to the theatre team, including the surgical (surgeon and scrub nurse), anaesthetic (anaesthetist and operating department practitioner) and post-operative care unit teams and then back to the ward. At each stage there needs to be a clear

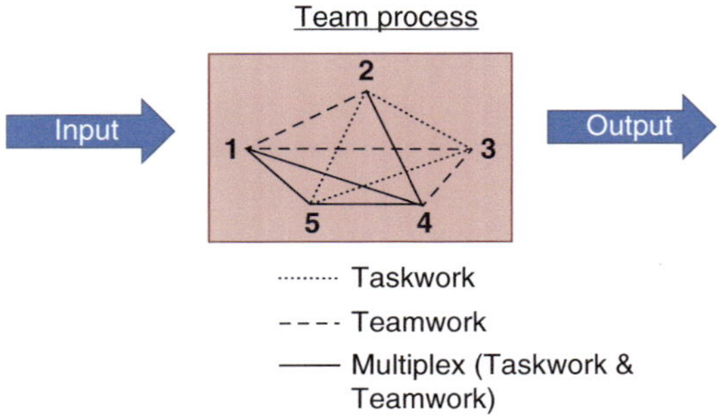

Fig. 9.1 Aspects of team process. Adapted from Crawford and Levine [6]

Table 9.1 Team activities. After West [9]

Team to organisation	Organisation to team
• Ambassadorial	• Targets
– Vertical interaction	• Resources
• Task coordination	• Informations
– Horizontal interaction	• Education
• Scouting	• Feedback
– Up to date information on external environment	• Technical/process assistance

handover of the patient between teams, an interface where even a simple breakdown in communication [10] has clear risks for patient safety (e.g. around wrong site surgery). These risks are well recognised and have been addressed through the theatre checklist, a World Health Organisation (WHO) initiative that has been introduced internationally, including in the United Kingdom (National Patient Safety Agency [11]) and SBAR (situation, background, assessment, recommendation) which has been introduced to aid verbal and written communication between medical teams [12]. These tools become particularly important when the patient's pathway is less well defined than that of a child with appendicitis and more like Jane's case where the clinicians involved, nursing and medical, may have never or only rarely been in a similar situation before.

As we have seen, communication between clinical teams is essential to optimise patient care but may be unfavourably influenced from within and between team biases. These biases can result in favouritism being shown to those within the team alongside prejudice against other teams who are stereotyped negatively with behaviour developing that may include limited information sharing [9]. One example of this was the midwifery team in Morecombe Bay Hospital in the U.K. who were described by Kirkup [13] in his report on the failures of the midwifery unit, as having an 'all for one' attitude and who '[pursued] normal childbirth "at any cost"'. This team of midwives worked together as a silo in an environment of poor relationships between clinical teams which led to 'repeated instances of failure to communicate important clinical information about individual patients'. When problems did arise the response was 'grossly deficient, with repeated failure to investigate properly and learn lessons'.

As we have seen communication within and between teams is a core activity for any team. Research by Pentland and colleagues [14] has shown that the pattern of communication between and within teams is the most important predictor of a teams' success across working environments. Using a methodology called Sociometrics, whereby a 'badge' worn by members of the team collects data on face-to-face interactions, conversation (including time talking, listening and interruptions), physical proximity and activity levels, Pentland showed that 35% of the variation in team performance can be accounted for by the number of face-to-face exchanges amongst team members. In addition, he described high performing teams as having a tendency to look outwardly and to 'oscillate' between this outward (exploratory) view and internal engagement to integrate any lessons learnt from the external perspective.

9.3 Team Training and Effectiveness

The question then arises as to whether any of these aspects of teamwork can be taught and if they can, what difference will improvements in team effectiveness make within a healthcare setting. Will improved effectiveness make a difference to patient safety?

There is a body of evidence to suggest that improvements can be made in team performance in various settings. Salas et al. [15] undertook a meta-analysis that included 45 studies, with 93 effect sizes representing 2650 teams of which 1660 were from labs or classrooms, 762 from the military, 138 aviation but only 80 from the medical sector. His analysis found that there was a moderate positive effect between team training and team cognitive, affective, process and training outcomes. However, these effects were moderated by educational content, team size and team stability. In particular, intact teams were noted to have the greatest benefit from training on performance outcomes when compared to ad hoc or more fluid teams (correlations of 0.49; 0.41–0.56 versus 0.31; 0.26–0.36 respectively).

Team training has been put into healthcare through programs such as TeamSTEPPS which concentrates on areas such as communication and team leadership [16]. The program promotes SBAR and other communication aids to promote communication between teams alongside 'effective team leadership' and 'mutual support', which help in breaking down hierarchies and improving internal communication. Improvement in these areas should improve team performance in ways that are measurable through improved patient safety, including morbidity and mortality.

A recent literature review [17] of 34 studies looking at improvements in patient safety found that six of nine studies that had mortality as an outcome measure, showed an improvement with training whilst 28 studies showed a positive improvement in patient outcome relating to other aspects of patient safety including improved morbidity. However, these studies were diverse in study design, interventions and outcomes measured. Only two of the studies were randomised controlled trials, neither blinded, whilst nine studies used cluster controls and the majority (23 studies) used an internal control. Further, many of the studies used other interventions alongside team training such as standardised protocols for specific tasks and the introduction of patient safety champions. Where studies had followed up the interventions, they showed that there was deterioration in performance once the intervention had stopped. This could be prevented by on-going training suggesting that resources, including team training, need to be maintained to ensure that improvements are kept and a cycle of improvement is developed (Fig. 9.2).

9.4 Fluid Teams

At this stage we need to consider once again the team that cared for Jane during the initial phase of her treatment. This team is a good example of a 'fluid team', one that changes over time, but maintains its common goal, in this case the care of Jane. The team was initially made up of staff from the ED but this began to change as the seriousness of Jane's illness was recognized. The pediatricians were called and a little later, the anesthetists whilst within these groups the more junior members called their seniors for support. Consequently, the team was constantly changing both in structure and leadership as those with differing expertise and seniority arrived. As the structure and leadership of the team changes, the transfer of relevant information to new team members alongside the ability of those taking on the leadership role becomes increasingly important to maintain a coordinated approach to care [19].

It is clear that the team caring for Jane needed to be adaptable to meet the changing demands placed upon it as the seriousness of Jane's condition was recognized and the level of treatment she received escalated. The team members needed to 'utilize their pooled resources … to adjust their actions according to situational requirements' [20]. Training of these teams needs therefore to concentrate on adaptability and shared understanding of roles including that of leadership.

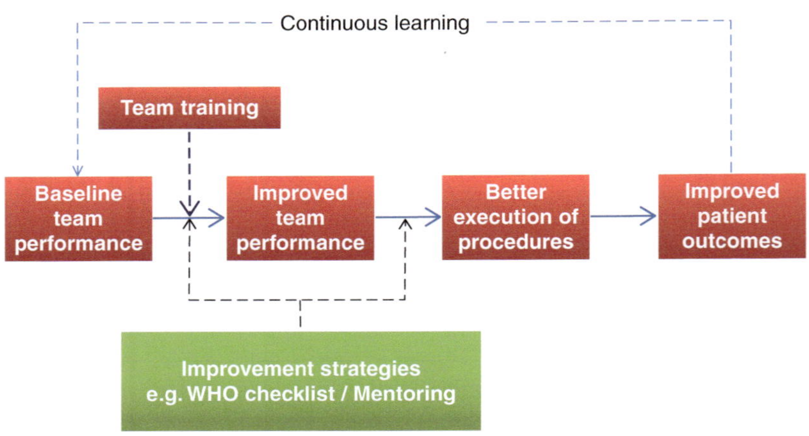

Fig. 9.2 The relationship between team training, teamwork and outcomes. Modified from Sorbero et al. [18]

Lewis et al. [21] have shown the benefits of teams training together through their development of 'transaction memory systems' (TMS) whereby individuals within the team have a greater understanding of each other's strengths and weaknesses and develop shared mental models of the situation faced and the functions of each team member. For fluid teams this TMS was maintained even when only some members of the team had trained together. This is important because fluid teams, by their nature, can usually only be defined in terms of roles rather than individuals for example, an anesthetic specialist trainee may be part of the clinical team but will also be part of the team of anesthetic trainees who make up the on call rota. The same will be the case for every role so that the chances of being able to predict the actual members of the team during training will be nearly impossible. However, what needs to be predictable is the ability of each team member to be competent to perform the task work assigned to their role, e.g. the anesthetist being able to intubate the child, even though he or she would not normally look after children.

This team training can take place through the simulation environment where rare but high risk clinical situations can be practiced in safety. Burke et al. [20] described a cycle of team adaptation requiring four phases; situational assessment, plan formulation, plan execution and team learning that can be practiced within simulations enabling rapid progression of fluid teams that themselves can be changed with each scenario.

9.5 The Organisation of Teams

So far we have considered the team working from a team rather than an organisational point of view. Hospitals, alongside most mature organisations, have traditionally been modelled on a vertical or hierarchical, structure so that individual teams work side by side feeding into divisions or directorates and upwards towards the executive. Within this structure efficiency has consistently been gained using the principles of scientific management first developed by Taylor and subsequently built upon by other methodologies such as the production line of Henry Ford, Japanese 'continuous improvement' and Deming's 'total quality management' [22].

However, for many clinical teams, this is an artificial, managerial, construct that takes no account of the patient pathways through the organisation that we have already considered. Although many of these interactions will be predictable, as will inter-departmental interactions in other organisations, others will be more complicated as they parallel the complexities of individual patients such as Jane.

These interactions and the consequences of failure make healthcare organisations more complex with both managerial and patient focused aspects creating tensions within the organisation (e.g. where does the financial cost of a treatment prescribed by one team and given by another lie?). In addition, workers and often leaders within the clinical teams are 'knowledge workers', university trained specialists who are 'dedicated to their careers and their specialities, not to their employers' [10] and therefore do not have the same loyalty to the organisation and willingness to work within the structure of that organisation. The first priority of these clinicians is the patient not the employer and the culture of their teams will parallel this.

These clinical teams can be managed along traditional lines but their ability to adapt to the changing healthcare environment will be limited. Other models need to be considered such as those described by General Stanley McChrystal and John Kotter. General McChrystal et al. [23] commander of the Joint Special Operations Taskforce in Iraq from 2003 developed a novel approach to organisational structure in response to the difficulties the task force were having in responding to the increased complexities of insurgency in Iraq having trained for more traditional military conflicts. Forces needed to adapt rapidly to ever changing situations and in order to achieve this, networks of teams were developed which enhanced resilience and the ability to organically reconfigure to meet new demands placed upon them. The outcome was a 'team of teams' which improved outcomes through improved communication and trust between teams.

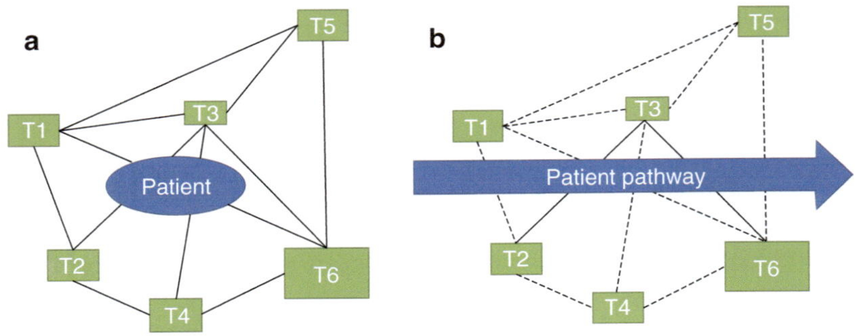

Fig. 9.3 Networks. (a) Patient centred network. (b) Network reflecting patient journey

This use of corporate networks has not been limited to the military. Kotter [24] noted that most companies during their start-up use a network based approach which then matures into a more traditional hierarchical structure. He questioned whether these traditional hierarchies could meet the rapidly changing demands of the modern business world and suggested that for mature companies to meet and grow within the additional complexities of modern business they needed to put into place a network alongside their traditional, hierarchical structure to produce a 'dual operating system' which was flexible enough to provide innovation and leadership to the organization.

There are clear parallels between the situation faced by McChrystal, the start-up organizations described by Kotter and the modern healthcare environment with its complexities of patients care, organizational structure and resource limitations. The question arises as to whether similar networks can be put into practice within the healthcare setting and in doing so what effect these lessons would have for patient safety? The concept of networks has been considered by the National Health Service in the United Kingdom both in the development of Strategic and Operational Delivery Networks as part of the changes introduced in response to the 2012 Health and Social Care Act [25] and more recently in the NHS 5-year Forward View [26] which described 'networks of care' to '[integrate] different organisations and services around patients'.

However, the networks described in healthcare, whilst patient centred may themselves become static structures that fail to meet the demands placed upon them (Fig. 9.3a). Rather, these networks need to be more dynamic and fluid in structure, recognising that patients, such as Jane, move through and between hospitals on a journey (Fig. 9.3b). Linkages between teams therefore need to be dynamic to reflect the multitude of journeys that can be taken.

One further aspect that needs to be considered is leadership. McChrystal et al. [23] described his team of teams but central to it working was the senior leadership he provided to drive through the changes required and embed them within the system. He saw his role as one of providing a 'holistic, big picture view' not that of micromanaging using a more reductionist approach. Kotter [24] took the importance of leadership further making clear that it was not just senior leadership that was required to develop and maintain a network but leadership at all levels within the organisation to mobilise the workforce towards change because 'there is no way that a single figure or small team at the top of the hierarchy can provide all the leadership that is needed'.

9.6 Summary

Jane survived her illness because the teams caring for her worked effectively. They adapted to meet her needs and coordinated with each other to smooth her journey.

For hospitals the challenge is for all teams, in every circumstance, to work effectively. Effective team working can be improved through training alongside other interventions although continued training is required to maintain the improvements made. Particular emphasis should be placed on fluid teams and their adaptability through methods such as simulation.

Networks of teams have been highlighted in healthcare but how they work effectively is still open to discussion and more radical network structures may be required to enable hospital teams to be adaptable to the changing healthcare environment. Any changes need to put patients at the centre of their structure but in a dynamic and responsive way.

For hospital teams to be effective they need to be adaptable to the needs of patients like Jane rather than expecting Jane to fit into an existing team structure.

References

1. Baker DP, Gallo J. Measuring and diagnosing team performance. In: Salas E, Frush K, editors. Improving patient safety through teamwork and team training. New York: Oxford University Press; 2012.
2. Kohn LT, Corrigan JM, Donaldson MS. To err is human. Building a better healthcare system. Washington, DC: National Academy Press; 1999.
3. Makary M, Daniel M. Medical error – a leading (but hidden) cause of death. BMJ. 2016;353(8056):237.
4. Baker DP, et al. The relation between teamwork and patient safety. Boca Raton, FL: CRC Press; 2011. p. 185–98.
5. Agency for Healthcare Research and Quality. TeamSTEPPS®: strategies and tools to enhance performance and patient safety. (2016). [online]. http://www.ahrq.gov/professionals/education/curriculum-tools/teamstepps/index.html
6. Crawford ER, Lepine JA. A configural theory of team processes: accounting for the structure of taskwork and teamwork (Report). Acad Manag Rev. 2013; 38(1):32.
7. Runciman B, Merry A, Walton M. Safety and ethics in healthcare: a guide to getting it right. 1st ed. Aldershot: Ashgate; 2007.
8. National Quality Board. Human factors in healthcare. 2013. [online]. https://www.england.nhs.uk/wp-content/uploads/2013/…/nqb-hum-fact-concord.pdf
9. West MA. Effective teamwork: practical lessons from organizational research. 3rd ed. Oxford: Wiley-Blackwell; 2012.
10. Johnson AB. The secret of Apollo. Baltimore, Maryland: The Johns Hopkins University Press; 2002.
11. NPSA (NPSA/2009/PSA002/U1). WHO Surgical Safety Checklist - NPSA/2009/PSA002/U1. London: National Patient Safety Agency; 2009.
12. NHS Institute for Innovation and Improvement. SBAR-situation-background-assessment-recommendation. (2008). [online]. http://www.institute.nhs.uk/quality_and_service_improvement_tools/quality_and_service_improvement_tools/sbar_-_situation_-_background_-_assessment_-_recommendation.html.
13. Kirkup B. The report of the morecambe bay investigation. The Stationery Office: Norwich; 2015.
14. Pentland A. The new science of building great teams: the chemistry of high-performing groups is no longer a mystery. (Spotlight on the Secrets of Great Teams). Harv Bus Rev. 2012;90(4):60.
15. Salas E, et al. Does team training improve team performance? A meta-analysis. Hum Factors. 2008;50(6): 903–33.
16. AHRQ (Agency for Healthcare Research and Quality). Pocket guide TeamSTEPPS 2.0. Rockville, MD: Agency for Healthcare Research and Quality; 2013.
17. Perring J. Teamwork, culture and patient safety. MBA Dissertation, Sheffield Hallam University; 2016.
18. Sorbero ME, et al. Outcome measures for effective teamwork in inpatient care: final report. Santa Monica, CA: RAND Corporation; 2008.
19. Summers JK, Humphrey SE, Ferris GR. Team member change, flux in coordination, and performance: effects of strategic core roles, information transfer, and cognitive ability (Report). Acad Manag J. 2012;55(2):314.
20. Burke CS, et al. Understanding team adaptation: a conceptual analysis and model. J Appl Psychol. 2006;91(6):1189–207.
21. Lewis K, et al. Group cognition, membership change, and performance: investigating the benefits and detriments of collective knowledge. Organ Behav Hum Decis Process. 2007;103(2):159–78.
22. Gallos JV. Organization development: a Jossey-Bass reader. Chichester: Wiley; 2006.
23. McChrystal S, et al. Team of teams. New rules of engagement for a complex world. Portfolio/Penguin; London, UK, 2015
24. Kotter JP. Accelerate: Building strategic agility for a faster-moving world. Boston, MA: Harvard Business Review Press; 2014.
25. The Health and Social Care Act. 2012 (Chapter 7).
26. NHS England. Five year forward view. NHS England. 2014. https://www.england.nhs.uk/ourwork/futurenhs/nhs-five-year-forward-view-web-version/5yfv-exec-sum/

What Is Change?

10

Silas Gimba

10.1 Introduction

Every day, healthcare systems cater for populations around the world and have ambitions of delivering safe, evidence-based care, without inequalities. The WHO estimates 234 million surgical operations are performed globally every year whereas, in the UK alone, hospitals provide health care for 1 million people every 36 hours. The turnaround of a failing hospital can be complex, costly and can cause long lasting reputational damage. Hospitals need to become adaptive and proactive, embracing change as a continuum by engaging with patients and other stakeholders in the change process.

Global healthcare systems and their hospitals are subject to powerful social and political influences. For example, opposing political philosophies of the two US political parties has driven the American healthcare system into a lingering state of transition with the uncertainties of 2010 Affordable Health Care Act ('Obamacare') likely to continue for years to come. Organised healthcare delivery in the US will remain in the flux created by the contrasting Democrats' philosophy of 'Big Government' versus the opposing Republicans' philosophy of free choice and free will.

In the UK, the National Health Service (NHS) has been a protected department since inception with all political parties. However, political influence is continually exerted on the NHS to reduce health costs and achieve an elusive balance between low cost and high quality of healthcare. Consequently, incidents of quality failures in UK hospitals have heralded substantial reforms or reorganisations in the NHS.

External influences significantly affect a health system's ability to deliver care at the time of need. With the risk of hospitals failing, this is a constant threat for those working in, managing or running hospitals, creating the reality that change has become a way of working life in healthcare. However, change is likely to be successful and sustainable if a hospital engages its doctors and supports medical engagement and leadership from within the organisation [1]. Medical engagement is one of the key factors preventing hospitals failing and this has achieved global consensus that this is a key element to achieve a successful healthcare system [2]. However while this has been a critical success factor to implement a paperless Electronic Patient Record for an NHS Hospital in the UK [1] a lack of a Trust wide culture of a medical engagement and leadership strategy is likely to increase the hospital's risk of failure.

S. Gimba
Obstetrics and Gynaecology, Diana, Princess of Wales Hospital, Grimsby, Lincolnshire, UK
e-mail: sgimba@me.com

P. Godbole et al. (eds.), *Why Hospitals Fail*, DOI 10.1007/978-3-319-56224-7_10

10.2 Change Is Inevitable

'No condition is permanent.'

Anonymous African Cliché

No situation, good or bad lasts forever, and we will all experience change. Benjamin Disraeli (also accredited to Heraclitus, Greek philosopher) is quoted to have said: "Change is the only constant". Disraeli is saying that the one certainty in life is that situations do not perpetually stay the same and change always happens, sooner or later.

When hospitals fail, quality of care deteriorates, and patients suffer avoidable harm: hospital associated infections, surgical misadventures, hospital falls and unplanned readmissions. There is a 1 in 300 chance of a patient being harmed during health care (World Health Organisation). Moreover, the UKs Care Quality Commission (cqc.org.uk) and US' CMO (www.medicare.gov) have all reported significant failings and low-quality ratings that traverse many of their best-known hospitals. Critical services such as cancer care, mental health services, maternity and emergency care suffer shortfalls. Waste and inefficiencies arise from lengthy stays, unplanned readmissions, duplicated or fractured service and litigation cost all of which compound intrinsic cost pressures.

10.3 Change in Hospitals Can Be Challenging

Quality Improvement (QI) requires a change in one form or another. Any turnaround, whether it is on a small scale such as reducing waiting list using PDSA cycles or a large, organisation-wide transformation using Total Quality Management (TQM) frameworks requires effective change. NHS England UK, is mandated to deliver the government's objectives for healthcare transformation for NHS England. The UK government's goal is to lead a step change in the NHS to prevent ill health; help create safe, high-quality health and social care services and balance the NHS' budget [3].

However, attaining a change in hospitals can be complex and challenging resulting in both unintended as well as intended outcomes. The relationship between change and progress is a tenuous one, after all, 70% of all transformational efforts fail [4, 5].

Successful organisational change is possible but often requires investment into a managed process, systems thinking and effective leadership. To be successful, today's leaders need to anticipate change and fully understand the principles of change and transition management [5, 6].

Organisational change requires effective affirmative leadership that starts with an understanding of what change is. Without an understanding of the inevitability of change and its complexity, leaders and managers risk unpreparedness during evolving circumstances. Leaders who fail to embrace socio-political influences or the heightened patient and public expectations from new technologies and advancing pharmaceuticals risk irrelevance.

The external factors that enforce change are generally outside the remit of a typical hospital manager's influence. Turnaround and positive change must come, therefore, from within. Given this, a critical skill set for leaders and managers in any major public, private or social enterprise is a grounded understanding of Organisational change [7].

10.4 What Is Change

'Change' is a term used commonly in general, business and management writings but there is a lack of conformity in both its application and context. The broad use of the term 'change' often equates to a move from a current state to a future state.

The transitive verb 'Change' is understood to mean 'make or become different' (Oxford and Webster dictionaries) and encompasses situations that alter, vary, modify, switch or transform. Because of the various interpretations of the term 'Change', academic writers typically refer to 'Change' in an Organisational context rather than the personal or individual context. Furthermore, simple daily operational management activity within organisations is not termed 'change'.

Change used in the organisational context refers to situations or events such a new structures, procedures, strategy or paradigm shifts but all characterised by the emergence of a different direction. The Society for Human Resource Management defines Organisational change as making things different by 'adopting corporate strategies, structures, procedures and technologies to deal with changes in external conditions and the business environment'.

10.4.1 Change vs. Transition

Change requires you to adapt to a new set of rules whereas, 'transition' is about these human impacts of organisational change and the psychological aspects of behaviour adjustment. Although change and transitions link closely in meaning, each describes unique perspectives of the change process.

Change is an 'event' that is visible and tangible. These events generate a variety of impactful psychological reactions among individuals or organisational teams: stress, anxiety, apathy and confusion. Bridges [6] defines Transition as how the change processes feel to the stakeholders or the internal processes that organisations undergo as they adapt to new events.

10.4.2 The Bridges Transition Model [6]

William Bridges was the first to model into three stages the differences in the speed at which individuals go through a transition. A transition starts with an ending.

Endings
Characterised by the need to let go and acceptance of loss. There is denial, disbelief and shock that may progress into resentment and resistance. Stress can be high.

Neutral Zone
The neutral zone is typified by when the 'old' has gone, but the organisation is yet to establish the new ways. Consequently, progress stalls, events become unclear and actions disordered.

Beginnings
Beginnings is when the new way feels comfortable, right and the only way. You make gains by establishing new behaviours, procedures and processes. There is a feeling of inclusion with an attachment to the new processes and systems.

10.4.3 Why Change Efforts Can Be Hard

Beckhard and Harris [8] were first to emphasise the need to manage the transition. Their Change formula state that to ensure a successful change, factor in the level of dissatisfaction with the status quo, create a vision of what you could achieve and know what first decisive steps to take towards attaining a change.

$$\text{Change} = [\text{Dissatisfaction} \times \text{Vision} \times \text{First steps}] > \text{Resistance}$$

Change is possible if the product of dissatisfaction (D), vision (V) and the first steps (F) is greater than resistance (R). Given that D, V, and F are multiplied, if any of these three is absent or low, then the product will be weak and incapable of overcoming the resistance.

Invariably, organisations that overcome resistance and manage change thrive while those that do not, struggle to survive.

10.4.4 Change Agents

Stakeholders have some form of interest in the change, whether they are the targets of the change, managers or other interested parties. The needs and expectations of the different stakeholders may conflict or influence change. There are three categories of stakeholders. Internal stakeholders (the workforce) are connected intimately to the organisation, and their objectives are likely to affect the change processes strongly. Connected stakeholders have a contract with the organisation such as customers (e.g., hospital patients), alternative suppliers or newcomers (e.g., independent private hospitals). External stakeholders include the governments, local authorities or groups with varying abilities to ensure the organisations meet their objectives.

A change sponsor is an individual with the ultimate responsibility to legitimise the change. A change agent is a person from inside or outside whose task it is to effect change or help an organisation get back on track with change management. An agent must be adept at communication, negotiation and managing their personal credibility. They must have influence within the organisation. Battilana and Casciaro [9] conducted studies of 68 change initiatives over 12 months in the NHS. Analysis of the networks of the middle and senior change managers showed that change agents who have interconnected networks are more efficient at implementing transformational changes. Network interconnection, therefore, is more effective for a change agent than formal seniority in a health organisation.

10.5 Personal Change

Being aware that change is unavoidable can help individuals anticipate shifts in their current situations. People respond differently to change, and that may vary from letting change happen, making it happen, resisting or disengaging from the process.

'Sometimes the things we believe about ourselves make it harder to accept change. So much so that you might deny the fact that change is happening at all.'

Who moved my cheese—John Spencer Johnson [10].

Adapting to personal change, therefore, requires self-awareness. Individuals' propensity for change is in part influenced by their belief systems, learning styles, behavioural, social and psychological makeup including the inclination to conditioning by rewards and punishments.

Change curve models such as adaptations of the Kubler—Ross Grief cycle [11] have thus, emanated from social and psychological theories. How individuals respond and adjust to change is not too dissimilar from Kubler-Ross' description of the psychological stages terminally ill patients undergo when coming to terms with their diagnosis. Denial, anger, bargaining, depression, acceptance and later experimentation with discovery typify a change framework.

The Myers-Briggs Type Indicator (MBTI) [12] is one of the several tools used to identify reactions to change in self and others by facilitating personal reflection. When it comes to change; different people bring in their individual MBTI preferences whether they are initiating the change or being influenced to undergo change.

Situational awareness can help people respond to change promptly and appropriately. Situational awareness is being aware of a developing situation around you, risks and threats that could result in difficulties in the short or long term. Acute situational awareness in the NHS forms the core attribute of NHS' Patient Safety measures such as the surgical safety checklists and perioperative team briefings. Long-term, to cope with changes leaders need situational awareness to avert the difficulties of a changing environment. Above all, to thrive, leaders and managers need self-awareness with an introspective mindset that permits adaptation to a changing work or life environment.

10.6 Group and Team Change

Team working is invaluable to a health care organisation. Experience in the UK health sector has shown a direct positive relationship between team working and organisational performance [13]. By definition [14], teams have a unified purpose, are dependent on their varied skills and pool information to enable them to accomplish individual goals.

Hospitals consist of a mix of skills and professionals and theoretically, should build high-performing teams. World Health Organisation's (WHO) data shows that one in ten patients may be harmed from adverse events such as hospital-acquired infections or errors such as medication errors while receiving care in hospitals [15].

A team approach is necessary to deliver safe surgery and so, a hospital's operating theatre team, for instance, consist of surgeons, anaesthetists, operating theatre nurses, theatre technicians, managerial and administrative staff all with uniquely distinct roles and skill sets. The WHO's patient safety fact files show surgical care errors contribute to a significant burden of disease even though, 50% of complications associated with surgical care are avoidable.

NHS staff survey data show staff incorrectly consider themselves working in real teams when these are pseudo-teams or groups. Of significance is the same data revealed that the higher the levels of staff working in pseudo-teams, the higher the level quality failures [16].

Salient interpersonal competition between individuals and interprofessional competitions between professional groups is not often apparent, and conflicts inherently arise within groups or teams of organisations [17]. That may in part, explain why the UK Department of Health's root-cause analysis of adverse events consistently show that barriers to the team working in hospitals may be rooted in inter-professional communication failures.

Additionally, real teams are 'mutually accountable' for their outcomes. However, professional allegiances, professional priorities and a misunderstanding or overlapping of interdisciplinary roles can impact negatively on teamwork in health care settings [18] and thus, adaptiveness to change.

The Belbin's team role model is a self-perception inventory for team members based on the work of Meredith Belbin that can help team members better understand their preferred roles in a change management situation [19]. For example, Implementers turn decisions and strategies into definable and manageable tasks, sorting out objectives and pursuing them logically. Implementers have proficient organisational skills with a good sense of what is feasible. This inclination favours competent management roles. However, the Implementer has the flaw of being uncompromising and resistant to change.

Using tools such as the Thomas-Killman conflict mode instrument [20] change managers can evaluate how differently individuals and teams respond to conflicts and peoples' preferred conflict management modes.

10.7 Organisational Change (Fig. 10.1)

Anderson in 1986 described the three most prevalent types of changes organisations undergo as developmental, transitional and transformational [21].

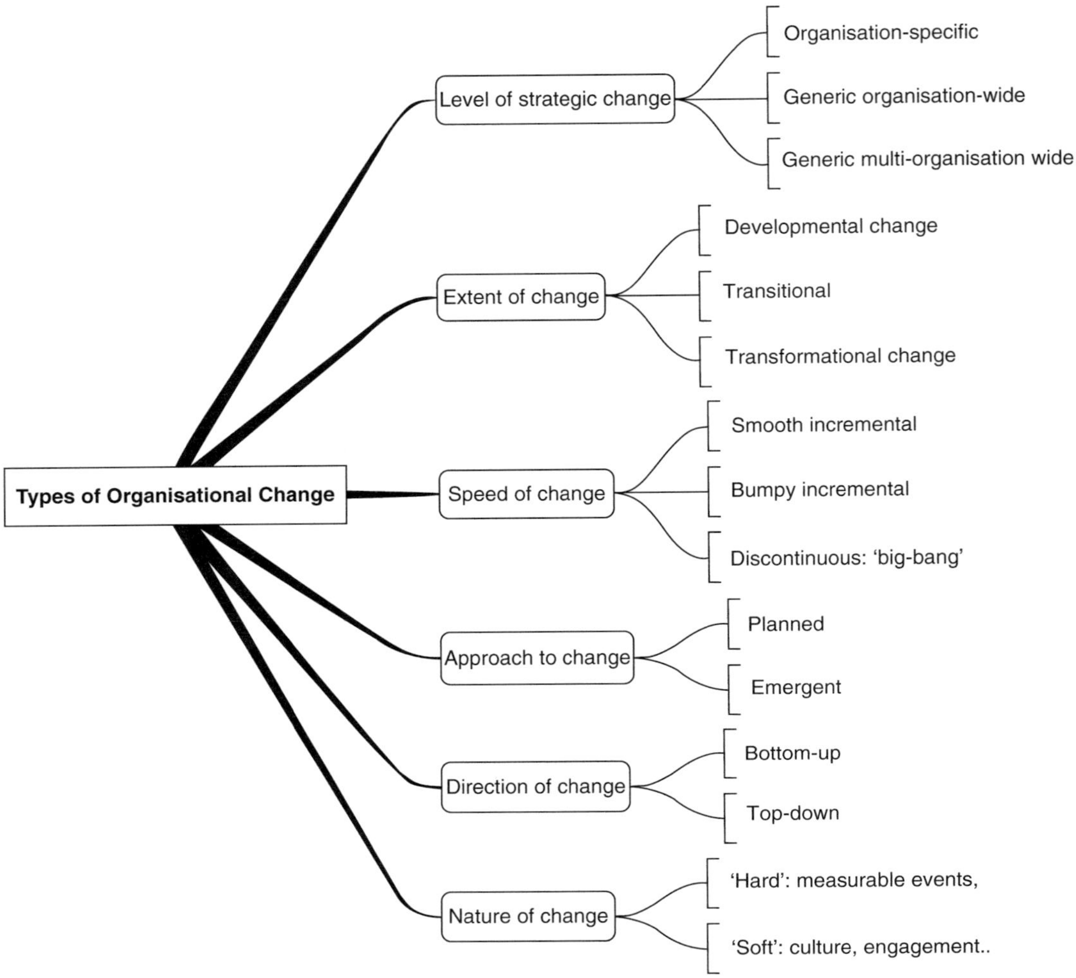

Fig. 10.1 Types of organisational change

10.7.1 Developmental Change

Developmental change improves performance continually through realignments to the existing situation while remaining within the confines of the same culture, structures and existing business practices. Developmental change may occur either through a series of adaptive workflows to realign a drifting strategy or a parallel of initiatives aimed at reconstructing the organisation.

10.7.2 Transitional Change

Rather than effecting improvements, a transitional change programme seeks to fix a problem through controlled incremental changes until the attainment of the desired state. This change model does not focus on culture but rather, 'hard' projects, structures and practices.

10.7.3 Transformational Change

Transformation seeks to establish a radically different situation that entails a cultural shift described figuratively as 'a caterpillar-to-a-butterfly' transformation where there is no going back. External factors wholly enforce the transformations that often require a change to survive or thrive.

Transformational change often occurs large-scale, and multi organisation-wide, in response to a decline in performance. For example, the NHS' 'biggest priority' in its 5-Year Forward Plan is to transform care outside hospitals. Note, however, the NHS regularly uses a transformational approach even for smaller scale changes in organisation-wide, continuous quality improvement projects, for example, the devolved Digital Revolution that seeks to transform care with fully interconnected electronic health records.

More often transformation is unplanned and may create a turbulent environment that is not necessarily within the control of leaders and managers. Balogun and Hailey [4] describe two subcategories of transformation: the 'evolutionary' change that is gradual and, in a big-bang transformation that is 'revolutionary'. Such transformative changes are more likely enforced with multiple initiatives occurring simultaneously [22]. Successful transformational change depends heavily on leadership.

10.8 Drivers of Change

Successful organisations continually strive to fill any gaps between what they deliver and what is likely to be required in the coming years (competitive advantage). Thus, the public sector like the NHS primarily aims to build or consolidate activities, its value stream, that maintain its core goals and to avoid strategic drifts. However, the NHS needs transformational change if it is to meet its founding objective of health for all from 'cradle-to-grave.' Subsequently, the NHS' value stream is grounded in The NHS Plan (2000) and most recently in the NHS' 5 Year Forward View documents [23] (Fig. 10.2).

External forces, internal factors or, as is usually the case, a combination of both trigger and influence change. The source of the change initiative, may, for example, be an externally legislated change where organisations may have little control over.

Change managers explore external environmental factors by applying the PESTLE (Political, Economic, Social, Technological, Legal, Environmental) analysis tool. PESTLE make up the 'opportunities or threats' in a SWOT (Strengths, Weaknesses, Opportunities and Threats) analysis. Thus, whereas strengths and weaknesses are internal organisational factors, opportunities and threats are external factors to influence change.

Internal factors, however, are internally conceived and planned change which is designed to exert some form of control aimed at achieving performance outcomes [7].

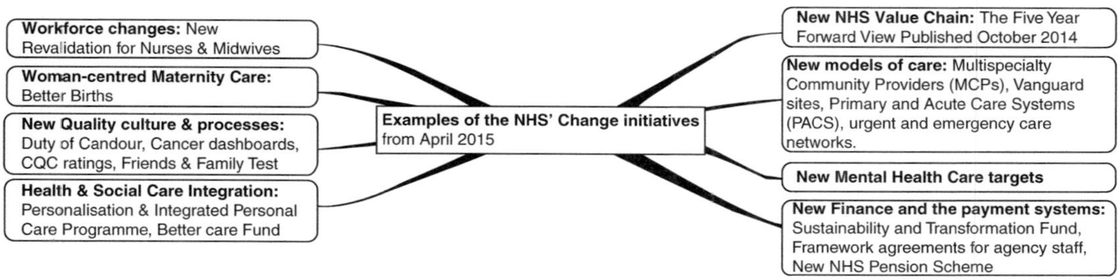

Fig. 10.2 Examples of the NHS' change initiatives from April 2015

Push and pull factors often combine to determine Organisational change. Push factors are the environmental forces that induce a change in the bid to survive. On the contrary, pull factors allow leaders longer views to consider the possibilities offered by surrounding opportunities, and the organisation has a choice. Porter's Five Forces is a management tool that places these factors into a framework to determine an organisation's ability to undergo change.

10.9 The Role of Organisational Culture and Change in Hospitals

Cultural assumptions and beliefs can aid or hinder changes that organisations are trying to make [24]. Hospitals have a mix of subcultures that impact on both individual and team behaviours and outcomes. These subcultures learned from past experiences of the group members are then considered valid enough to be taught to new members as the 'way things are done here'.

Hospitals often proclaim, 'the patient comes first', but in reality, the other priorities overtake this consciously espoused belief. Thus, the normative culture of hospitals may be 'patient-centred', ultimately an active sub-culture that is bureaucratic and hierarchical intervenes. This dominant hierarchical culture in hospitals values stability and structured control.

Misalignments between the normative and the real cultures impact negatively on the process of Organisational change. Gidden's structuration theory and the 'duality of structure' throw some light into such conflicting social systems. Clinicians value evidence-base and are guided by a sense of professional autonomy that is embedded in their training. Professional autonomy (i.e. the Gidden's structure) either constrains or enables the actions of clinicians (the agents) even if this runs in sharp contrast to that of other agents such as managerial or non-clinical staff. Managers have a structure that is not constrained or motivated by professional autonomy but by administrative accountability for quality and efficiency.

Consequently, hospital managers and senior hospital clinicians have by nature, different motivations and professional values. This lack of understanding of what motivates the other is a constant source of conflict between leading hospital doctors and managers. The Gidden's duality of action explains actions of senior doctors and what they legitimise as right or wrong. These measures become self-perpetuating through which they communicate or exert power.

Change in hospitals, therefore, can be difficult in part because to effect transformative change, change managers need to close this gap between these current and preferred cultures, and this takes knowledge, skilled effort and time.

10.10 Change Management

Change differs from change management. The Society of Human Resources and Management (SHRM) define change management as the systematic approach and application of knowledge, tools and resources to deal with change. Change management means: setting and adopting corporate strategies, structures, procedures and technologies to address changes in external conditions and the business environment www.shrm.org.

One of the earliest tools of change management was Lewin's three-phase change management model that focused on the transition.

1. Unfreezing
   - Prepare the organisation for change by recognising and accepting the need for change and the undesirability of the present situation. Unfreezing serves to lower resistance and creates the initial motivation to change.
2. Movement (Change)
   - Movement is the change itself when you help people embrace new attitudes, behaviours and culture that develop into the new norms.
3. Refreezing
   - Refreezing is establishing the stability and support systems to maintain the change event. It is reinforcing the new pattern of work or behaviour as the new reality e.g. by rewards systems.

No approach to change is perfect and there is no one-size-fits-all approach to change management. Methods can be integrated. Other tools worth applying are the Kotter's eight step change model, McKinsey's 7-s Model, Beer's model, Rodgers' Diffusion of Innovators and ADKAR organisational change management tools. Regardless of how you approach change, identifying the key stages involved in the change process increase the likelihood of making better-informed decisions. That is, making decisions about which interventions to use to overcome resistance, create a vision with buy-in and, effect or adapt change.

10.11 The Role of Change Leadership

Northouse [25] defines leadership as a process whereby an individual influences a group of people to achieve a common goal. Northouse's definition is multifaceted and implies 'process'', 'influence', 'group dynamics' and a 'unified goal.' Change leaders have the capacity to steer people by using their personal attributes and behaviours to accomplish the desired change.

Change leadership matters to an organisation undergoing change since cultural changes cannot happen without leadership. Change leaders help followers to tackle and effect change from a position of conflict and the realities of their situation [25].

The challenge for hospitals is acquiring the personnel with these required skills and qualities. To avert failed change leadership, Eckert et al. [26] argue for diversity in the leadership of hospitals to a majority with clinical backgrounds.

Eckert et al. [26] argue further for a collective leadership style that enables continual quality improvements, staff engagement and talent acquisition. That is rather than the common NHS' organisational focus on meeting targets, budgets and maintaining corporate policies.

For the often overworked, under-resourced clinicians in hospital management, the challenge is alternating between active participation and reflective observation [27, 28]. The term 'hybridity' has been used to explain how clinicians maintain a professional identity as physicians while taking on management responsibilities [28, 29].

Much less has been researched on hybridity with the development of medical leadership as opposed to medical management functions; however, the literature on hybridity draws upon social identity theory to show how doctors may seek to maintain their social identities as physicians while undertaking non-clinical tasks and activities. Removing ambiguity from medical leadership tasks provides a useful framework to define the actions of leadership. Such functions are providing direction, influencing followers through their ideas, values, meanings, providing emotional and cognitive support and, inspiring by providing good examples.

In conclusion, the impact of politics, globalisation, economics and new capabilities from technological innovations drive stakeholder needs and expectations. Behavioural and cultural shifts is an inevitable fact of life for the individuals, groups and teams that make up and run health organisations. These transformational changes require effective leaders and managers with skills to anticipate strategic drifts yet, understand and value the human aspects of transition and change processes.

References

1. Gimba S, Aylott J, Kilner K. The UK National Health Services paperless vision and the challenges of clinician engagement and leadership: evaluative case study of an acute secondary care hospital. In: The 5th annual global healthcare conference (GHC), Singapore, 18–19 July 2016.
2. Baker RG. The roles of leaders in high performing health care systems. Kings Fund Publications; 2011. kingsfund.org.uk.
3. Department of Health. The mandate: a mandate from the government to the NHS Board. 2013. Available at www.gov.uk/dh.
4. Balogun J, Hailey VH. Exploring strategic change. Upper Saddle River, NJ: Pearson Education; 2008.
5. Kotter JP. Leading change why transformation efforts fail. Harv Bus Rev. 2007:92–107.
6. Bridges W. Managing transitions: making the most of change. 3rd ed. London: Nicholas Brealey Publishing; 2009.
7. Rees G, French R, editors. Leading, managing and developing people. 4th ed. London: CIPD Publications; 2013.
8. Beckhard R, Harris RT. Organizational transitions. 18th ed. Reading: Addison-Wesley Publishing Company; 1977.

9. Battilana J, Casciaro T. The network secrets of great change agents. Harv Bus Rev. 2013;91(7–8):62–8, 132.
10. Johnson S, Blanchard KH. Who moved my cheese? Spencer Johnson. London: Vermilion; 2015.
11. Kübler-Ross E. On death and dying. New York: Collier Books; Toronto: Maxwell Macmillan Canada; New York: Maxwell Macmillan International; 1993.
12. Briggs-Myers I, McCaulley MH, Quenk NL, Hammer AL. MBTI manual: a guide to the development and use of the Myers-Briggs type indicator. Palo Alto: Consulting Psychologists Press; 1998.
13. Steward K. Staff engagement: six building blocks for harnessing the creativity and enthusiasm of NHS staff. London: The King's Fund; 2015. Available at: http://www.kingsfund.org.uk/sites/files/kf/field/field_publication_file/staff-engagement-feb-2015.pdf. Accessed Oct 2015.
14. Katzenbach J, Smith D. The wisdom of teams. Brighton, MA: Harvard Business Review Press; 2015.
15. World Health Organization. WHO 10 facts on patient safety. WHO. 2014. Available at: http://www.who.int/features/factfiles/patient_safety/en/. Accessed Nov 2016.
16. West MA. Creating a culture of high-quality care in health services. Glob Econ Manage Rev. 2013;18(2):40–4.
17. Mullins LJ. Management and organisational behaviour. 11th ed. London: Pearson Higher Education; 2016.
18. Nason F. Diagnosing the hospital team. Soc Work Health Care. 2008;9(2):25–45.
19. Belbin RM. Team roles at work. 2nd ed. Abingdon: Routledge; 2010.
20. Thomas KW. Thomas-Kilmann conflict mode survey. Tuxedo; 1974.
21. Anderson D, Anderson LA. Beyond change management: how to achieve breakthrough results through conscious change leadership. San Francisco: Wiley; 2010.
22. Johnson G et al. Exploring strategy: text and cases. 11th ed. Harlow: Pearson Higher Ed; 2016.
23. NHS Five Year Forward View. "NHS England." Public Health England, Monitor, Health Education England, the Care Quality Commission and the NHS Trust Development Authority. NHS England. Five-year forward view; 2014.
24. Schein EH, Schein P. Organizational culture and leadership. 5th ed. Wiley: Hoboken; 2016.
25. Northouse PG. Leadership: theory and practice. 5th ed. Thousand Oaks: Sage; 2010.
26. Eckert R et al. Delivering a collective leadership strategy for health care. London: The King's Fund. 2014. Available at http://media.ccl.org/wpcontent/uploads/2015/04/DeliveringCollectiveLeadership.pdf. Accessed Oct 2015.
27. Heifetz RA. Leadership without easy answers. Cambridge: Harvard University Press; 1994.
28. Joffe M, Davey KM. The problem of identity in hybrid managers: who are medical directors? Int J Leadersh Public Serv. 2013;8(3):161–74.
29. Spyridonidis D, Hendy J, Barlow J. Understanding hybrid roles: the role of identity processes amongst physicians. Public Adm. 2015;93(2):395–411.

11 Why do People Resist Change?

Prasad Godbole

11.1 Introduction

We have seen from the previous chapter that change is inevitable and is a constant feature in our lives. Whether it is an ongoing step wise change to make an existing state better (a developmental change [1]) or a dramatic transformational change [2], it is here to stay. The two extremes of change can be very clearly highlighted in our lifetime. The progression of telephones from the dial phones, to analogue through the digital age of mobile technology is a classic example of a developmental change. The current political climate in the USA and a new President elect has led people to a state of not knowing what is going to happen and this can be considered to be a transformational change. By the time this book is published however, the USA population will have entered into a new phase of equilibrium following the transformation. Which change would one consider to be the more accepted by people? In the vast majority I would suggest it is the developmental change [3]. This chapter will not dwell on the change per se but on why people resist change. I will try and provide examples of my experience of people resisting change. The subsequent chapter will give the next contributors personal perspective and experience on overcoming change.

P. Godbole
Department of Paediatric Surgery,
Sheffield Children's NHS Foundation Trust,
Sheffield, UK
e-mail: Prasad.Godbole@sch.nhs.uk

11.2 Factors Causing Resistance to Change

There are many factors that can contribute to individuals resisting change. It is imperative for leaders to identify and empathise with these factors to be able to overcome this resistance. In many hospitals globally, the management structure is led by non clinical managers [4]. How many times has it been noted that change has been attempted only for it to be shelved as being unsuccessful [5]? In most of these instances, the clinical front line staff are blamed for the failing of the change [6] rather than the non clinical managers lack of insight into the pitfalls in change management [7].

Fear We are all creatures of habit and more regimented than most in the healthcare sector. We are used to arriving to work at a certain time, getting our morning coffee from the same place at the same time every day, meetings, lunch, and then clocking off at the same time. We all have our designated roles and responsibilities in the work place and get paid for this work undertaken. However when a change is debated there is always a discussion about the need for change. Why fix something that isn't broken? is the common phrase heard. This is because there is a distinct unease about

P. Godbole et al. (eds.), *Why Hospitals Fail*, DOI 10.1007/978-3-319-56224-7_11

what the advantages are for the proposed change, compared to the way things are now. Will I lose out financially? Will my working pattern change to a more performance managed work schedule? Will I still have a job? All these fears [8] can be allayed by continued and ongoing dialogue at an early stage and a transparency about the rationale and need for change. Good leaders manage this process by engagement and getting buy in from the champions from the group they work with. In the U.K. the junior doctors strikes over terms and conditions of weekend working is a prime example of fear on the part of the junior doctors on what the new contract would mean to them but also suggests a lack of dialogue throughout the process to prevent these strikes.

Loss of Control Maslow's hierarchy of needs [9] provides a framework to explain how our needs are presented in a hierachy or order of needs dependent on the status of our physiological, emotional and psychological needs being met. According to Maslow, those higher up in terms of seniority of role in the organisation have already usually achieved their lower order goals and leading a team is likely to meet Maslow's 'Esteem needs' providing a feeling of accomplishment and in many cases a feeling of empowerment. Imagine if the change being suggested involves reallocation of resources that challenges your feelings of self esteem? Not only do you stand to lose face with your team who you had previously led, but there may be implications for employment including secondment or loss of a job. This is more so in private organisations rather than the publicly funded organisations like the National Health Service in the United Kingdom. However, the transformation agenda for the NHS will impact directly on those senior in the organisation, now more than ever before.

Uncertainty of the Future Part and parcel of the transformational change is the uncertainty about the future [10]. A deck of cards has been thrown up in the air and no one knows how the cards will land. Let us take the example of the President Elect in the United States. His election was greeted with protests across the country by ordinary civilians. Why? Some feared a nuclear war, some feared far right groups would be able to dominate, others feared cultural and religious segregation. The fact of the matter is no one knows what will happen. Unless there is a period of time after the swearing in ceremony; it is impossible to know what the next 4 years will produce. When there is no certainty, this leads to fear, loss of control as described above. Eventually however no matter how the next 4 years progress, individuals reach a new steady state and a new equilibrium within the new state although this may not be perceived as good as the previous state.

Not Understanding the Rationale for Change One of the main reasons cited for dissent amongst the workforce to change is lack of communication around the reasons for the change [11]. If the workforce is unable to envision the rationale for the change, this then becomes an abstract notion of change. Poor communication and a top down approach to force through the change at the request of the senior executives is a key feature of unsuccessful organisational changes. Early dialogue, transparency, openness, empathy towards the individuals affected by the change and two way communication on a continual basis by effective leaders can overcome this resistance.

The Reality Is Painful Sometimes the reality of change can be stark and painful. In the context of patient safety, organisations have a mandatory duty to ensure that patients are treated in a safe and efficient and effective manner. Relevant safeguards to achieve this must be put in place and corners cannot be cut. Patient experience is paramount and the quality of care a priority. In the first chapter the editors discuss the relationship between finance, delivery, activity and quality/effectiveness. Hospitals may fail if they are unable to balance these factors and if patient safety deteriorates. In the U.K. the Care Quality Commission (www.cqc.org.uk) inspects both public and private hospitals as well as any healthcare provider against patient focused standards. An inability to evidence patient safety and outcomes against the standards prompts a poor rating and close monitoring. NHS Improvement (https://improvement.nhs.uk) is another organisation that looks at the overall viability of a hospital. In failing hospitals, the healthcare regulators e.g. Monitor and CQC may declare a hospital is in special measures. What change does this entail? Gone are the entire executive management team and replaced by an 'interim turnaround team'. This is a team recruited by the healthcare regulators and placed in situ for a period of time in the failing hospital. This is a reality and painful for all stakeholders as decisions will be made that may not be suited to the needs of the local context. The report 'An Organisation with a Memory' produced by the Chief Medical Officer, in the UK, 2000, advised that we must learn from adverse events and near misses that impact on patient safety. Producing an organisational learning culture within healthcare orgnisations requires clear and transparent whistleblowing procedures. The report suggests that whilstleblowing can be seen as a failure to learn "as people are far more likely to pursue chanels outside their own organisation if there has been a failure to act on or even acknowledge concerns raised internally" (p.64). Much better to invest in a positive communication strategy to support organisational change within a 'no-blame' culture and be supportive of different organisational interest groups.

Ripple Effects Let us continue with the example above. A hospital has been put in special measures and the executive management team replaced. Most of the middle tier managers and clinical and allied clinical staff understand that the hospital has failed in patient safety, poor quality, financially, and in the delivery of commissioned activity. All the previously discussed factors come into play. The new team are the turnaround team and so processes have to be put in place swiftly to ensure financial stability and sustainability of the organisation. This could lead to ripple effects within the transformational change process, including reorganisation of entire departments leading to loss of jobs, new ways of working, restructuring of roles and responsibilities with new job descriptions and pay scales. Leaders should be prepared for such an event and communication is key to ensure a smooth change process.

More Work An often cited reason for resistance to change is that it would create more work [8]. There is certainly a concentrated focus on elements of change that do need more work. However this is more work only if this is added on to an individual's work schedule. Good leaders would get the individual to focus only on the extra work as their sole work for the period of change and backfill their role on a temporary basis. An organisation had been aware of their lack of accurate coding of surgical procedures and therefore revenue generated was below the level expected. The surgical procedures were handwritten and the coding process was poorly coordinated and inefficient. A change to electronic data entry and drop down menus to populate the surgical procedural and diagnostic codes as well as co morbidities was instituted. The IT department felt that the amount of work required to undertake this change including teaching and training of the clinicians was too much for the capacity within their team. However allocating two members from their team to work with clinicians in theatres over a 6 month period allowed a smooth transition to the new system, better recording of data and improved coding.

Past Experience Individual personalities can form a barrier to change [12]. Because I do not like or get on with person x makes me oppose anything person x says. This may be because person x and I do not see eye to eye on a number of issues or especially at senior management level, there can sometimes exist a power struggle between executive members. Survival of the fittest can sometimes lead to individuals looking after themselves as the first priority and at any cost rather than looking towards improving an organisation. The consequences of such organisational behaviour when not held to account can result in bullying and harrassment of employees. A National Training Survey in 2013 (report by the General Medical Council) reported that over 13% of Junior Doctors reported being victims of bullying and harrassment in their training posts, with female doct ors who gained their primary medical qualification outside of the UK more likely to make a comment about bullying or undermining. The NHS Employers Association in the UK have identified that bullying and harrassment costs the NHS a significant amount in lost sick days, with respondents who have been bullied taking on average 108 days off work and a third have contemplated leaving their jobs (The NHS Employers Association, 2016; Johnson, S, 'NHS staff lay bare a bullying culture' The Guardian, 26 October, 2016).

Competence In many industries including hospitals, success is led by effective leaders as has been discussed in the preceding chapter on what is a leader and an effective medical leader. The ability to use various styles of leadership but also monitor and reflect upon the outputs from the leadership style, form an important part of the success. Lack of leadership can lead negatively to the same process spreading vertically downwards through the management structure. An organisation where there is no performance management or just done to tick a box can hide the true competence of individuals within the organisation. Change management can expose these individuals for their true skills and competencies against their job description and can lead to opposition if the individual has the insight to realise that with change their competence may come into question to perform the same task [12].

Conclusion

Change is inevitable, it will happen. Many factors cause people to resist change. Understanding these factors as they relate to the healthcare sector before change is contemplated is important. Leading change by effective medical leaders along with senior management rather than non clinical managers alone is also important (see Chap. 12—clinicians versus managers or the new hybrid).

References

1. Andrew H, Van de Ven V, Marshall SP. Explaining development and change in organizations. Acad Manag Rev. 1995;20(3):510–40.
2. Chapman JA. A framework for transformational change in organisations. Leadersh Org Dev J. 2002;23(1):16–25.
3. Weick KE, Quinn RE. Organizatinoal change and development. Annu Rev Psychol. 1999;50:361–86.
4. The Kings Fund. The future of leadership and management in the NHS: no more heroes; 2011. pp. 1–47.
5. Franklin JL. Characteristics of successful and unsuscesful organization development. J Appl Behav Sci. 1976;12(4):471–92.
6. Cooke HF. Scapegoating and the unpopular nurse. Nurse Educ Today. 2007;27(3):177–84.
7. Huq Z, Huq F, Cartwright K. BPR through ERP: avoiding change management pitfalls. J Chang Manag. 2006;6(1):67–85.
8. Kanter RM. Ten reasons people resist change. Change Management. Harvard Business Review. www.hbr.org. 2012.
9. Maslow AH. A theory of human motivation. Psychol Rev. 1943;50:370–96.
10. Torben R. Top 12 reasons why people resist change. Available at: http://www.torbenrick.eu/t/r/hwj. 2011.
11. Sridhar B. Common cause of resistance to change is lack of awareness. Available at: www.thehindu.com. 2011.
12. Agboola AA. Managing deviant behaviour and resistance to change. Int J Bus Manag. 2011;6(1):235–42.

Overcoming Resistance to Change: A Personal Perspective

12

Umesh Prabhu

Working out your core patient-centred values and communicating these values to colleagues is a critical role for the medical leader. Being able to influence upwards, across and through many related and inter-connected organisations is a challenge to ensure the spread of a patient centred, patient safety culture. So how might this be done? But before identifying *how* to influence and how to bring people with you on the change journey, it is important to know *what* to influence and for what purpose. It stands to reason that if everyone is working for the patient and everyone prioritises patient centred values, then this should provide the impetus and driver for change. But unfortunately this is not always the case as organisations are complex and multi-faceted, and change is never that simple. This chapter will draw upon my own personal values and influences that shaped my decision to enter into medicine as a Paediatrician while also drawing upon specific examples throughout my career as a doctor and more latterly as a Medical Director. I will identify the strategies that I have used to enable change in organisations, specifically where there have been examples of resistance to change. Values based leadership, based upon core values of respect, kindness, valuing fellow human beings and human dignity has enthused me to drive improvement in patient safety and enhance the patient experience for many patients in the NHS over the years.

12.1 Early Beginnings and Influences

Coming from a small village in India, my family values were a strong influence and so too was the drive to succeed. It was almost inevitable that I would study medicine as opposed to engineering as I was surrounded by role models who would emphasise morality and humanitarianism. My sister studied medicine but gender inequalities in rural India did not enable her to practice her passion, rather she reverted to an expected gender role of wife and mother. Her humbleness and compassion for others were ever present and I felt driven to accept the place at medical school that she had applied for on my behalf. The writings of Mahatma Gandhi were also shaping my destiny as a doctor and he believed "morality is the basis of things and truth is the substance of all morality". I wanted to be a good doctor and to never let children down.

In 1982, I followed a colleague who had come to the UK as a Doctor. I arrived in Yorkshire, newly married with great expectations but with a significant culture shock in a country that went dark at 4 pm and had snow! After passing my exams I applied for over 60 jobs and wasn't short

U. Prabhu
Wrightington, Wigan and Leigh NHS Foundation Trust, Wigan, UK
e-mail: palimar.prabhu55@gmail.com

P. Godbole et al. (eds.), *Why Hospitals Fail*, DOI 10.1007/978-3-319-56224-7_12

listed for one. Remaining positive, I reflected on this with my medical supervisor and eventually I managed to secure a locum post and then went on to apply for a job in Bury. The transition for an overseas doctor to adjust to the context of the UK is significant and I could not have made such a successful transition had it not been for the support of individuals along the way. In my new post in Bury, a very good registrar said to me "don't worry I am here for you". Those words resonate with me even now. The feeling of being guided and supported to practice medicine in a new country was the most powerful feeling at this time which made me aware of the importance of coaching and mentorship for the effective transition of medical practice for overseas doctors. It also reinforced the idea that feeling valued by others in the workplace was an extremely important aspect for leaders and managers to encourage. If we want to promote the valuing of patients, then we need to start by valuing our staff.

Throughout my career at this hospital and another in Scotland as a Registrar, there were individuals who would take me under their wing and guide me. The kindness and compassion of my work colleagues, often senior, sometimes brusque in their mannerisms were to highlight the importance of a compassionate work environment. Kindness in the workplace is the key to thriving and being motivated. Being kind and compassionate to others is critical in the engagement of colleagues who are "resistant to change". So often hospital managers default to "performance management" systems to manage people's behaviour by control and micro-management—yet it is the opposite of this that will support individuals to feel safe enough to consider change. But they will need mentoring and coaching to undertake a transition that they may feel difficult and challenging to them and they may not want to give up old behaviours. Acts of kindness and positive feedback can help others to feel valued and supported to make changes required in the workplace. As a senior medical leader, I try to send out positive emails to staff on a weekly basis to praise, support and engender feelings of value amongst the medical staff. It is also important to recognise that many of the skills of leadership and management are not taught at medical school. So often doctors are left to work out for themselves how to deal with difficult and challenging situations at work with individuals and teams. Leadership and management skills should be available to all doctors and not just considered as an optional extra for a few doctors. Such skills should be developed while developing systems improvement to advance patient safety.

I faced many challenges in practising medicine, but felt it was always right to be honest and truthful and to remember the things that are important such as being open to patients. Since the Mid Staffordshire hospital crisis [1, 2] the duty of candour has been promoted as critical to promote a safe and honest patient safety culture, but for many of us practising medicine it is part of the way we have always related to others and is a core value of our being and a core value of our medical training. Telling the truth and being honest makes us vulnerable but also makes us better doctors. Vulnerability can make us feel fearful and afraid that we must never make mistakes. But to 'err is to be human' as Don Berwick argues [3]. Human beings are likely to make mistakes, however it is down to us to develop systems to minimise errors and to reduce the risk and vulnerability of doctors. I try to learn from all of my mistakes and to support others to share in that learning. Back in 1992 we had two six week old babies, with the same names in the same ward. One baby was sent home without child protection checks as the wrong notes were checked after examining the baby. The baby sadly died at the hands of the step father and after a root cause analysis six things had gone wrong. We put in a system against each of these. In a report 15 years after the seminal report 'To Err is Human' [4, 5], there is a suggestion that we still have a lot to do to embed patient safety in our health systems. A revised checklist for safety improvement has been produced [4] (Fig. 12.1).

I had the opportunity to work as a senior registrar and researcher at Oxford with one of the world's leading researchers in paediatrics. This job took me across the country travelling to all Trusts and undertaking work to develop knowl-

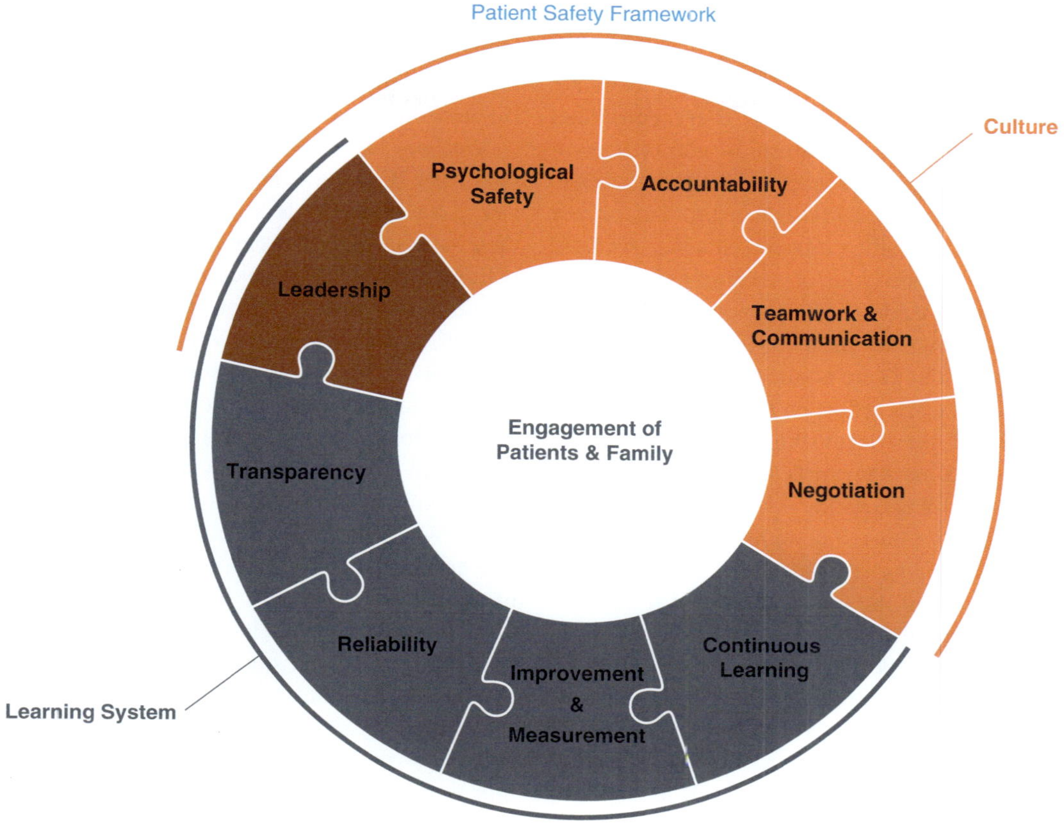

Fig. 12.1 A patient safety framework (source: Institute of Healthcare Improvement IHI, 2015)

edge and understanding of meningitis in children. I was also working on call at the Trust in Oxford, to continue to develop my experience as a doctor, which prepared me for a post as a consultant paediatrician in Bury. I ended up working back alongside my mentor and supervisor and developing a collaborative service between GPs and hospital doctors. It was through this integrated working that we generated a trusted and respected service with general practitioners who increased their referral rates from 800 to 1400 children in the course of a year. I have since learnt that it is the time invested in relationships with our colleagues in community practice that will generate further business for the Trust. I invested time to attend evening meetings with GPs and prioritised telephone calls for inquires and calls for help from GPs to invest in this relationship. Across the globe, the more successful hospitals will invest time for their hospital doctors to form relationships with their community counterparts and to build these relationships into a core part of their organisational strategy and business development. However this is not standardised practice across all hospital Trusts where doctors are 'job planned' in a finite way to deliver increased levels of activity to deliver the operational business rather than provided with a balanced job plan to include Quality Improvement and new service development. However, funding for healthcare in the National Health Service in the UK, through the tariff structure only funds operational business and not service improvement and business development. Michel Porter in his article 'the strategy that will fix health care' [6] argues that funding for service improvement needs to be available to make the transformation required in the NHS.

At the time when I was in post as a Clinical Director, it fell to me to undertake this more strategic role, yet the posts of Clinical Directors are too few in the organisation. Every consultant needs to formulate relationships with their community colleagues, to develop leadership skills to promote the quality services they provide to those who have the ability to refer patients. As Lord Darzi [7] visioned, doctors need to be clinicians, partners and leaders. However leadership development takes time while developing and applying new skills. There is often little thought as to how doctors will reflect on the impact and effectiveness of their leadership to promote patient safety. One mechanism is to support the use of Action Learning Sets [8] as a good forum to support doctors to have time to reflect on the quality improvement journey. This needs to be supported from the top of the organisation and recognised as an important feature of an organisation that is taking safety improvement seriously.

Working in a patient centred way is an extension of the core values of kindness in the workplace, happy staff will be positive with patients and want to improve the service. Unhappy staff will just come to work and see it as a job rather than as a vocation. I felt it important to communicate our core values to General Practitioners, to tell them how we work and how we valued patients. I told them that if a mother has no transport for her child then I will come to her. I told them that we will work together to learn from the times when things do not go well so that we can improve the services we offer to patients. We had to confront our biggest fears at these times and believe that these values contribute to an honest and open culture within a hospital setting. In 1993 another baby died at 36 weeks of age 16 hours after discharge from hospital. I took the notes home, to look at what went wrong. There had been a procedure that should have been undertaken by the doctor as soon as the babies temperature rose. This hadn't happened quickly enough with this baby. We knew that it was a continued risk to get a doctor to the baby immediately if there was a change in temperature, so I trained the nurses and developed the clinical governance protocol that was approved at the clinical governance board. I wanted to improve the system so that another baby did not die from the same fault in the health system.

Working in this way and within a team, will only work if all team members have the same values. I have always recruited medical staff for their values. If they have the right values then all compliance to Trust policies and the practising of medicine will be undertaken in a similar way by all staff. Values based staff will work to improve the service and strive for excellence. As a Medical Director in 1998 I set to work to challenge an organisational culture that had been formed and shaped on idiosyncratic personal preferences of individuals (clinical and non-clinical) across the Trust. Waiting lists had become part of the culture and there was no appetite to challenge some of the basic 'waiting list' thinking. Some of the old habits that had developed over time was due to a lack of agreed quality standardisation in delivering procedures. In the absence of a system to engage doctors in patient safety improvement and the development of quality standards, doctors were keen to be busy and to develop their clinical practice. For many doctors they switched their efforts and attention to the development of private practice. Without 'safely and kindly' challenging some of these old practices, there was no impetus for individuals to change. They would be likely to resist all change if it appeared to be a management instruction. We had to change the culture and raise our expectations of our doctors. We wanted doctors to lead on patient safety improvement initiatives and we had to find ways to enable this to happen. The error was in the system and not with the individual doctors. My own values based leadership approach encouraged others to look at systems improvement rather than to blame individual doctors.

There had been a lack of opportunity for clinicians to discuss quality throughput and to balance clinician time against the commissioned contract. I started a dialogue with clinicians about waiting lists in their clinical areas and we explored ways in which we might bring the waiting list down. There were some difficult conversations but we tried to focus on how we can gain system improvement rather than to focus on personalities. It was important to find the clinicians strengths and to align their competence with various clinical roles and commissioned work. This would build an effective team and enable collaboration as opposed to competition. Continual Professional Development days were used to help target the development of new skills. Some clinicians were not working to their strengths with some procedures taking them four times longer compared to their colleagues. However team job planning helped to discuss the abilities and strengths of colleagues who had become 'super specialist' in specific clinical procedures and who could undertake some procedures more effectively and efficiently than others. We reduced the waiting list in orthopaedics from 18 months to 11 months and specifically in arthroscopy we reduced the waiting list from 1.5 years to 1 year.

The NHS has had a history of 'pace setting' as a management and leadership culture, which is defined by Goleman [9] as when the leader sets extremely high performance standards and leads by example. This approach can overwhelm team morale, so too can the commanding style, whereas other styles such as coaching, visionary, affiliative and democratic promote harmony and positive outcomes [10]. Pace setting and being commanding is not a conducive style for improving a patient safety culture in any hospital and those with a dominant culture of this will see the hospital fail.

While waiting lists continued to be a challenge, there were also greater challenges facing the reduction of patient harm, improving patient safety and reducing mortality at the hospital. Shortly after being in post as a Medical Director, I identified 27 patients that had been harmed due to doctors practices. Preventable deaths is a critical point of learning for doctors and we must learn from every death. I started asking for the patient notes of every patient that had died and we started to take case notes home to examine what factors had gone wrong. Courage is the most important quality that is needed when we need to face our greatest fears. Knowing that doctors never intentionally come into work to harm patients, I needed the courage to understand how the system can cause premature and preventable deaths. My work at the National Patient Safety Agency supported me to champion the advancement of patient safety in the Trust and I was also National Clinical Assessment Advisor for the National Clinical Assessment Authority for a period of 15 years. Both roles have helped me to understand that without effective clinical governance systems and mentoring and support for doctors, doctors are often subjected to investigation about their practice. Fifty percent (50%) of doctors are not told they are under investigation and many suffer personal and long term tragic consequences when things go wrong.

Conclusion

With national shortages of doctors in many specialties and the risk of closure to some departments due to the shortage of clinical staff, we need to support doctors to develop in this fast changing context. Providing a supportive, values based culture, where clinical governance systems outline standardised quality criteria and leaders and managers are recruited for their values and use supportive leadership and management styles, is the way forward. We need investment in innovations of new ways of working, so that doctors can be inspired rather than experience fear. Inspiring and enthusing doctors will lead to greater levels of motivation a nd a patient safety culture.

References

1. Francis R. A report into the mid staffordshire hospitals inquiry. 2011.
2. Francis R. A final report into the mid staffordshire hospitals inquiry. 2013.
3. Berwick D. To err is human: building a safer health system. Institute of Medicine; 1999.
4. Berwick D. 15 years on after: to err is human: the status of patient safety in the US and the UK. 2015.

5. Illingworth J. Continuous improvement of patient safety: the case for change in the NHS. 2015.
6. Porter ME and Lee TH. The strategy that will fix health care. Harvard Business Review; 2013.
7. Maybin J, Thorlby R. High Quality Care for All. London: The Kings Fund; 2008. p. 1–11.
8. Revans R. The ABC of action learning. 2011.
9. Goleman D. What makes a leader: why emotional intelligence matters. Harvard Business Review Press; 2014.
10. Goleman D, Boyatzis R, McKee A. Primal leadership: unleashing the power of emotional intellegience. Harvard Business Review Press; 2002.

Organisational Learning 13

John Edmonstone

13.1 Introduction

This chapter considers what we might mean by an "organisation" and how learning takes place within it. Most employees of organisations will be mature adults, so an examination of how adults learn in work contexts is also addressed. The unusual nature of healthcare organisations, such as hospitals, is explored and the question of by what means such organisations can learn is examined and some major ways forward are suggested.

13.2 What do we Mean by an Organisation That It May Learn?

We tend to take organisations like hospitals for granted as the places where we work and spend much of our waking time, but we typically underestimate their ephemeral nature. Who remembers now such organisations within the National Health Service in England as Regional Health Authorities (RHAs), Area Health Authorities (AHAs), District Health Authorities (DHAs), Primary Care Groups (PCGs), Primary Care Trusts PCTs), Regional Offices (ROs)and the NHS Executive (NHSE), not to mention more currently Area Teams (ATs), Clinical Commissioning Groups (CCGs), NHS Trusts (NHSTs), Foundation Trusts (NHSFTs), Health and Well-Being Boards (HWBBs)and NHS England? They all seem to appear and disappear in a word-salad of "re-disorganisation", all of which makes for significant confusion.

At the root of this problem may be what can be termed the "positivist" viewpoint in the social sciences—that of treating all organisations as concrete entities with some kind of objective existence quite independent of those who work within them and those who seek to lead and manage them—and thus organisations such as hospitals are seen as easily definable and measurable [1]. This is a form of "reification" which occurs when human creations (which all organisations undoubtedly are) are misconceived as *"facts of nature, results of cosmic laws or manifestations of divine will"* [2].

We are therefore in real danger of ignoring vital organisational dynamics, particularly those relating to organisational politics and to emotion, as these are *"complex, difficult to understand and at times overwhelming"* [3]. From a quite different perspective organisational life can be seen to be co-created by both the rational **and** the emotional and so organisations are *"the temporary product of interactional processes"* [4]. This emphasis is much more on the social process of **organising** than on organisations as entities. This view therefore rejects the possibility of one objective "truth" or "grand narrative" in favour of

J. Edmonstone
Keele University, Newcastle-Under-Lyme, UK

MTDS Consultancy, Ripon, UK
e-mail: john.edmonstone@btinternet.com

P. Godbole et al. (eds.), *Why Hospitals Fail*, DOI 10.1007/978-3-319-56224-7_13

a reality that is socially constructed and in which context and culture both influence and are influenced by the actors in the scene who, in turn, shape and are shaped by this process and in which the worldview is constantly reformed and negotiated by coalitions and powerful players. No single independent and objective "organisational" truth can be known, because we (all of us) are participating in or co-constructing that process.

All organisations, including hospitals, are therefore far from being just rational, planned and stable entities. Organisational reality is fundamentally shaped by the conversations and dialogues that take place between the people within them and this, of course, is constantly shifting. From this perspective "organisations" are rather communities of meaning, sustained and perpetuated by communication and interaction patterns and shaped by individuals' power relations and emotions. Organisational learning is therefore the process of creating, retaining and transferring knowledge (in its' widest sense) within an "organisation" and between "organisations". It can therefore best be seen as a means of encouraging "systemic eloquence"—the ability of parts of a system (an organisation such as a hospital, a group of hospitals in a locality, a care network or a system) to talk well to each other [5].

13.3 What Is the Nature of Adult Learning?

Adult learning is now properly understood as an organismic or natural "living" process, rather than an ego-driven process [6]. This means that it is not something that "I" do, but it happens of itself, often in spite of "I" and not because of it. Learning is also not something confined to formal and structured settings such as educational and training programmes (academic or otherwise), but can also be informal in nature—that is, predominantly experiential and non-institutional—and may also be incidental—that is, unintentional and as a by-product of other activity [7]. We can therefore say that while individual human beings are naturally "programmed" to learn, organisations are not.

What is known in adult learning terms is that:

- ***Learning starts from not knowing:*** It is only when people honestly admit that they do not know how to proceed that they really become open to learning. There can be no experts in those situations in which there are no "right" answers and no obvious ways forward. Where there are no right answers then people must act in order to learn. Learning can be seen as sharing and exploring our ignorance.
- ***Learning involves the whole person***: People do not usually, in practice, separate their emotions from their intellect. The recent popularity of the concept of Emotional Intelligence is a clear recognition of the critical role that emotion plays in learning [8].
- ***Much learning is episodic in nature, rather than continuous:*** It seems to take place in short bursts of relatively intense activity which absorb the learner's attention and comes to an end when the immediate purpose of learning has been achieved. People then resort to a much slower pace of learning before the next intensive episode takes place, stimulated by a problem, situation or issue which demands resolution.
- ***We feel the urge to learn when we are faced with difficulties we would like to overcome:*** Real-world problems provide us with the motivation to learn. People who take responsibility in a situation have the best chance of taking actions that make a difference. We learn most, and best, when what and how we learn is experienced as relevant.
- ***Learning is not just about the assimilation of knowledge, but also about the recognition of what is already known:*** Learning is inevitably based upon, and builds on, previous experience. It involves both what is taught and also our questioning insight. It is not only the acquisition of yesterday's ideas but also the trying-out of new and unfamiliar ideas. It involves asking useful questions in conditions of uncertainty and therefore involves a degree of risk—taking actions that may or may not work.
- ***A powerful block to learning is our predisposing way of seeing the world:*** Our "mindset" or

way of seeing the world has inevitably been formed by previous experience and is made up of our fears, hopes, dreams, speculations, queries, hunches, intuitions, habits, identifications, unconscious projections, half-baked notions, prior training, social conditioning and internalised cultural expectations. These are typically not shared, explicit or even logical when viewed by others but they contribute to the patterns (of beliefs, traditions, fears, conflicts) that make some things possible and others impossible to each one of us.

- ***Revision of mindsets is easier in a safe and secure atmosphere:*** We learn best with and from other people as peers when addressing together those pressing difficulties to which no-one knows the solution. Learning is increased when we are asked questions by our peers and reflect on what we did; when we have time and space to address problems and when we are both encouraged, supported and challenged [5].

13.4 What Is the Nature of Healthcare Organisations?

The conventional wisdom has long been to evaluate and judge healthcare organisations such as hospitals in exactly the same way as other types of organisation. Yet there is a powerful case to be made that all healthcare organisations (but particularly hospitals) are fundamentally different from industrial and commercial enterprises and even from other organisations operating in the public sector. The closest parallels would be with people working in other "human service organisations" such as schools, colleges, universities, social services and the police [9] where "street-level bureaucrats" [10] historically have operated in conditions of high discretion and low prescription when dealing with the public. The reason for this difference is because the people who work in hospitals (particularly clinical staff) have to undertake what is termed "emotional labour". Emotional labour is a recent term used to describe a much older phenomenon. Revans [11] from work at Manchester Royal Infirmary originally described a hospital as an institution *"cradled in anxiety"* and Menzies-Lyth [12] highlighted healthcare staff as bearing:

> the full immediate and concentrated impact of distress, tragedy, death and dying which arise from patient care and which are not part of the typical working experience for most of the public.

while Tallis [13] identified that:

> It is easy to forget the appalling nature of some of the jobs carried out by healthcare staff day-in, day-out – the damage, the pain, the mess they may encounter, the sheer stench of diseased human flesh and its waste products.

and that:

> Contact with emotional distress and disturbance can be…harrowing. Existential questions about identity, suffering, madness and death are raised and may put people in touch with extreme feelings of confusion, pain and loss. The struggle with feelings of helplessness and hopelessness in the face of suffering cannot be avoided and individuals, depending on their personality and past experience, protect themselves in different ways from the emotionally traumatic environment

Emotional labour is therefore the *"suppression of feeling in order to sustain an outward appearance that produces in others a sense of being cared for"* [14]. An example of 'emotional labour' was illustrated in Chapter 2, where doctors were significantly 'emotionally' challenged in providing End of Life care to patients. Without a supportive infrastructure, the team had faced high levels of staff sickness. In practice 'emotional labour' involves:

- Depersonalisation and categorisation of hospital patients.
- The cultivation of professional detachment and self-control—a *"caring but distant"* demeanour vis-à-vis patients and relatives.
- Ritualistic task performance involving checking, rechecking and form-filling as avoidance.
- Delegation upwards to seniors in order to avoid responsibility.
- Suspicion of organisational change—or alternatively an obsession with regular reorganisations.

The protection against anxiety that care-giving induces by the suppression of personal emotions over a sustained time-period leads to a reduced ability to withstand the emotional toll of care which, in turn, leads to either burn-out or unhealthy detachment—no longer noticing or acting on the distress of others. These were, of course, features of the Mid-Staffordshire Hospital situation.

While this is true of individual healthcare workers and of healthcare professions, there is also a greater organisational impact:

> Healthcare organisations operate in society as "containers" of the emotions and anxieties of patients' relatives and families and because of this the experience of leaders and managers of clinical professional staff is different from that of an industrial/commercial enterprise. Managerial initiatives from the 1980s onwards have served to increase and bolster the potential defence mechanisms in play to deal with the inherent anxiety of working in healthcare. Increased bureaucratisation of professional work has also served to increase prescription and decrease discretion. [15]

As a result, learning in healthcare organisations such as hospitals is inevitably marked by the nature of the work undertaken by clinical professionals, but also permeates and influences the entire organisation [16]. There is a real danger that when a scandal such as that at the Mid-Staffordshire Hospital is exposed the default "solution" involves the imposition of further bureaucratic controls and even the mandating of formal education and training for staff—but these in themselves cannot guarantee individual, group and "organisational" learning or change in work practices.

13.5 How "Organisations" Might Learn

A concept that may be useful in considering how systemic eloquence might be enhanced is that of **absorptive capacity**—the capacity of an "organisation" to acquire assimilate and apply knowledge. Absorptive capacity is shaped by both external and internal factors. The former include:

- Wider environmental conditions experienced by a hospital, such as the pace of change or the scale of challenge faced.
- How easy it is for a hospital to access both explicit and tacit knowledge about performance and how that knowledge is shared and transferred at all levels and across all staff groups.
- How a hospital works with other stakeholders (such as local authorities, the private and voluntary sectors) and whether those relationships exhibit a high degree of collaboration, trust, mutual respect and parity, and how close or distant these relationships are.

The latter comprise:

- How inward-looking or outward-looking a hospital is—how it responds to experimentation and innovation in both clinical and managerial terms
- How hierarchical or controlling it is.
- The existence of strategies that make the focus of hospital performance improvement clear, are shared and supported by all staff groups and are realistic and consistent.
- The existence of intra-hospital structures and processes for enacting the mobilisation of knowledge—activities such as intelligence-gathering, capacity development, change management, etc.

The way that hospitals acquire, assimilate and apply such knowledge (or in other words learn) seems to be shaped by a combination of these external and internal factors [17]. So how might such learning be fostered? A number of major strategies have been developed. These are:

- ***Action Learning Sets***: *Action learning is "a method for individual and organisational development based upon small groups of colleagues meeting over time to tackle real problems or issues in order to get things done, reflecting and learning with and from their experience and from each other as they attempt to change things."* [18]. Action learning sets can operate within an organisation such as a hospital, across several organisations and even across an entire health and social care system [5]. Obolensky [19] asserts that most organisations are stuck in a charade because those at the "top" know that they do not know the answers to the questions facing the organisations that they lead—but feel that they *should* know—and so pretend to know. Likewise, those at the "bottom" do know most of the ways forward and also know that people at the "top" do not know, yet they expect them to know, and so they often pretend not to know! As Revans, the instigator of action learning said allegedly *"Doubt ascending speeds wisdom from above"*. The action learning approach in healthcare has been particularly linked to whole-system change conferences. Dialogue and collective engagement was mobilised between a number of such sets ("a structure that reflects") and large change conferences—a space where reflection could be linked to power ("A structure that connects") [20]. Such a process requires the active engagement of key hospital decision-makers in order to ensure success, echoing Gentle's [21] imperative for the need for senior decision-makers to move beyond mere rhetoric. Similarly, Olsson et al. [22] highlighted the importance of early time and effort being devoted to trust-building across professional boundaries and emphasised the importance of such factors as support from senior management, the modelling of openness, the need to agree codes of conduct or rules of engagement and the need to meet at a "neutral" venue.

- ***Large Group Events:*** A whole range of approaches and techniques have been developed under this heading. These approaches give as much importance to the understanding and resourcefulness of participants as to those of subject-matter experts. Participants reveal to themselves and to each other their own experience, beliefs and mental models. For this to happen, time and space are needed in which individuals can engage in conversations through which their mental models may change. The overall mix of participants (and thus the wide variety of perspectives) is key here. The approaches include:
  - ***Conversational Conferences*** [23]: These are designed to engage participants' practical experience and interaction with external experts in order to promote conversations and networking that works and also to promote implementation after the event. This is pursued through focus on a shared task, topicality, opportunities for mutual support and question and answer.
  - ***Future Search*** [24]: This is the most structured of the large group approaches with the primary purpose typically being system-wide strategic planning. It is particularly applicable when enabling diverse (and possibly conflicting) groups to find common ground for constructive action and new approaches to address "wicked" problems [25] A long lead-time, preparation through a steering group composed of representatives of the various stakeholders and an event of three days duration are all necessary. Part of the purpose is to get representatives of the whole system into the room and working together.
  - ***Open Space*** [26]: A more fluid version of some of the other approaches.
  - ***Real-Time Strategic Change*** [27]: Similar to Future Search, but capable of dealing with larger numbers of people. There is also a focus on building and maintaining a common database, fostering a sense of community and identifying preferred futures.

These approaches have a growing track-record of application in the public sector, including healthcare, world-wide and within the UK.

- In addition, there are a number of well-established and pre-existing methods and approaches already in use in hospitals and which enable the sharing of information, experience, perceptions, etc between individuals, professions and groups. They include:
  - ***Teamwork development***: Increasingly it is realised that much healthcare can only be delivered by professional and multi-

professional teams, and this is particularly the case in the hospital setting. While there is a tendency to mis-label any grouping of staff (even groups as large as 20 people) as a "team", they are better described as "pseudo-teams". Nonetheless, there is evidence of emerging good practice in team working in healthcare, and especially in hospitals [28].

- ***Benchmarking:*** This involves seeking-out and implementing best practice at best cost across several hospital organisations, selected on a like-for-like basis, as a means of comparison [29].
- ***Coaching and mentoring***: These are the most widely-used development methods employed globally in all kinds of organisations and have an emerging track-record of success in healthcare and increasingly with hospital staff, especially when directed towards situations of conflict or the need to work across professional and/or organisational boundaries [30].

The whole point, however, is that these should not simply be "initiatives" either inspired locally or imposed nationally, but should be part of a comprehensive and well thought-out local approach to developing absorptive capacity within the hospital which is sensitive to the local setting or context, considering such matters as local culture, history and so on.

Conclusion

Our understanding of "organisations" has fundamentally changed from seeing them as concrete entities to regarding them as communities of meaning. Mature adults working in healthcare organisations such as hospitals learn best when addressing pressing problems in the company of their peers. Hospitals are unlike other types of organisation because of the emotional labour which is part of the lived experience of clinical staff. Absorptive capacity offers a conceptual model for viewing organisational learning and the encouragement of systemic eloquence can be facilitated through a wide variety of approaches, provided they are designed and delivered as part of a well thought-through approach to developing absorptive capacity locally within the hospital setting.

References

1. Francis H. HRM and the beginnings of organisational change. J Organ Chang Manag. 2002;16(3): 309–27.
2. Berger P, Luckmann T. The social construction of reality: a treatise in the sociology of knowledge. New York: Anchor/Doubleday; 1966.
3. Vince R. Action learning and organisational learning: power, politics and emotion in organisations. Action Learn Res Pract. 2004;1(1):63–78.
4. Rigg C. Action learning for organisational and systemic development: towards a "Both-And" understanding of "I" and "We". Act Learn Res Pract. 2008;5(2):105–16.
5. Edmonstone J. Action learning in healthcare: a practical handbook. London: Radcliffe Publishing; 2011.
6. Claxton G. Wholly human: western and eastern visions of the self and its' perfection. London: Routledge & Kegan Paul; 1981.
7. Marsick V, Watkins K. Lessons from informal and incidental learning. In: Burgoyne J, Reynolds M, editors. Management learning: integrating perspectives in theory and practice. London: Sage; 1997.
8. Goleman D. Emotional intelligence: why it can matter more than IQ. New York: Bantam Books; 1996.
9. Edmonstone J. Human service organisations: implications for management and organisation development. Manag Educ Dev. 1982;13(3):163–73.
10. Lipsky M. Street-level bureaucracy: dilemmas of the individual in public services. New York: Russell Sage Foundation; 1980.
11. Revans R. Standards for morale: cause and effect in hospitals. Oxford: Oxford University Press; 1964.
12. Menzies-Lyth I. The functioning of social systems as a defence against anxiety: a report on a study of a nursing service of a general hospital. In: Menzies-Lyth I (1988) editors. Containing anxiety in institutions: selected essays. vol. 1, London: Free Association Books; 1959.
13. Tallis R. Hippocratic oaths: medicine and its' discontents. London: Atlantic Books; 2005.
14. Hayward R, Tuckey M. Emotions in uniform: how nurses regulate emotions at work via emotional boundaries. Hum Relat. 2011;64(11):1501–23.
15. Edmonstone J. What is wrong with NHS leadership development? Br J Healthc Manag. 2013;19(11): 531–8.
16. Hinshelwood R, Skogstad W, editors. Observing organisations: anxiety, defence and culture in health care. London: Routledge; 2000.

17. Walshe K, Harvey G, Skelcher C, Jas P. Could do better?: knowledge, learning and performance improvement in public services. Swindon: Manchester Business School/University of Birmingham, Economic & Social Research Council; 2009.
18. Edmonstone J. The action learner's toolkit. Aldershot: Gower Publishing; 2003.
19. Obolensky N. Complex adaptive leadership: embracing paradox and uncertainty. Farnham: Gower Publishing; 2014.
20. Nicolini D, Sher M, Childerstone S, Gorli M. In search of the "structure that reflects": promoting organisational reflection practices in a UK Health Authority. In: Reynolds M, Vince R, editors. Organising reflection. Ashgate: Aldershot; 2004.
21. Gentle P. The influence on an action learning set of affective and organisational cultural factors. Act Learn Res Pract. 2010;7(1):17–28.
22. Olsson A, Wadell P, Odenrick P, Bergendahl M. An action learning network method for increased innovation capacity in organisations. Act Learn Res Pract. 2010;7(2):167–79.
23. Pratt J, Plamping D, Gordon P. Conversational conferences: from ideas to action. Br J Healthc Manag. 2003;9(3):98–103.
24. Weisbord M, Janoff S. Future search: an action guide to finding common ground in organisations and communities. San Francisco: Berrett-Koehler; 1995.
25. Rittel H, Webber M. Dilemmas in a general theory of planning. Policy Sci. 1973;4(1):155–9.
26. Owen H. Tales from open space. Potomac: Abott Publishing; 1995.
27. Jacobs R. Real-time strategic change. San Francisco: Berrett-Koehler; 1994.
28. West M, Lyubovnikova J. Illusions of teamworking in health care. J Health Organ Manag. 2013;27(1):134–42.
29. Ettorchi-Tardy A, Levif M, Michel P. Benchmarking: a method for continuous quality improvement in health. Health Policy. 2012;7(4):101–19.
30. West M, Kirsten-Armit L, Eckert R, West T, Lee A. Leadership and leadership development in health care: the evidence-base. London: Faculty of Medical Leadership & Management/Centre for Creative Leadership/Kings Fund; 2015.

14 Learning to Lead: Tools for Self Assessment of Leadership Skills and Styles

Ann L.N. Chapman and Prosenjit Giri

14.1 Introduction

There is now general acceptance of the importance of engaging physicians in leadership roles [1, 2]. It is recognised that strong clinical leadership can improve a range of important outcomes within health services [3–6]; and conversely that lack of clinical leadership and engagement contributes to poor quality of care and patient outcomes [7–9]. Leadership development for clinicians has been promoted through national initiatives such as Darzi Leadership Fellowships for doctors in training and the national NHS Leadership Academy ([10–12] 'Leadership and engagement for improvement in the NHS'). In addition to national developments, the Smith review [5] concluded that more decentralised and locally designed leadership development programmes are required.

Despite this focus on medical leadership development, there remains little understanding of the optimal way of 'teaching' leadership skills to clinicians, most programmes typically using a positivist approach of transfer of theoretical knowledge with little attention to building self-awareness [13]. Furthermore there has been very limited evaluation of outcomes: where outcomes have been examined these have been limited to outcomes at the individual rather than at team or system level [13]. The optimal balance of taught versus experiential learning is unclear: do developing leaders need to be given the opportunity (with support) to experiment, indeed to fail, in order to grow in knowledge and wisdom? Medical leaders vary widely in clinical and personal backgrounds, and in leadership and management training [14], and the optimal balance between general content versus that tailored to the specific needs of the individual is also unknown. If tailored, how do we determine individuals' learning needs? There are a number of leadership assessment tools but few have been rigorously tested in the area of medical leadership, particularly in relation to the validity of self-assessment.

There is no doubt that a key requirement for effective leadership development at the level of the individual medical leader is self-awareness. This will be innately present to varying degrees in individual leaders but can be enhanced and increased through structured reflection on one's own personal experiences [15] and also through observation of the leadership of others. Self-awareness can also be increased through the use

A.L.N. Chapman (✉)
Monklands Hospital, NHS Lanarkshire, Glasgow, UK

University of Glasgow, Glasgow, UK
e-mail: ann.chapman2@nhs.net

P. Giri
Sheffield Teaching Hospitals NHS Foundation Trust, Sheffield, UK

University of Sheffield, Sheffield, UK
e-mail: Prosenjit.giri@nhs.net

P. Godbole et al. (eds.), *Why Hospitals Fail*, DOI 10.1007/978-3-319-56224-7_14

of self-assessment tools, although paradoxically such tools may be less reliable in people whose self-awareness is low. Self-awareness allows identification of strengths and weaknesses, and allows an individual to focus their personal development more effectively.

In this chapter we review two examples of the use of self-assessment tools in medical leadership. In the first, we focus on the paradigm of leadership styles, that is, not *what* the leader does but *how* he or she leads, using two complementary models of leadership styles. In the second example, self-assessment of leaders' own leadership skills is undertaken around the seven domains of the NHS England Leadership Academy Healthcare Leadership Framework [29]. The same framework can be used in other healthcare organisations globally.

14.2 Study 1: Self-Assessment of Leadership Styles Used by Senior Medical Leaders

The concept of leadership style relates to the behaviour of individual leaders; Pennington [16] defines leadership style as 'the behaviours and habits that individuals use to influence and manage people'. Over 400 individual leadership styles have been described, illustrating the difficulty in defining the true basis of leadership effectiveness. However there are some common underlying principles, for example, that individuals use a small number of styles preferentially, and that effective leadership is associated with use of styles appropriate to the given setting.

In this study two models of leadership styles were used [17]. The first model comprises six leadership styles based on aspects of emotional intelligence [18] (Table 14.1). These styles were derived from a global study of over 3800 business executives looking at specific behaviours and their effects on organisational climate, assessed through factors such as sense of responsibility to the organisation, clarity about the mission and values and freedom to innovate [18]. The authoritative style had the most positive impact on organisational climate, followed by

Table 14.1 Descriptions of leadership styles (adapted from [19])

Affiliative	Promotes good relationships and communication within the group. She/he is interested in the personal welfare of her/his team members. She/he gives positive feedback frequently yet may be uncomfortable giving negative feedback. Some team members may feel that she/he should be more forceful and provide clearer direction to the team.
Coaching	Concerned with supporting the efforts of others on the team and developing their skills. She/he helps team members to identify their strengths, weaknesses and potential, provides ongoing performance feedback and sees mistakes and underperformance as learning opportunities. However, the focus on individuals may limit the productivity of the team as a whole.
Commanding	Provides clear direction and expects others to follow. She/he is comfortable making quick decisions with little input from others, and excels in a crisis. She/he does not hesitate to confront others when they are underperforming, but rewards those who excel in their work. She/he is less skilled at listening to others' ideas and some team members may feel demotivated and lose enthusiasm.
Democratic	Encourages participation and exchange of ideas from her/his team. When faced with a complex problem, she/he will elicit ideas from others, listen attentively and build consensus, but may put off making difficult decisions. Some team members may feel that she/he should "decide" more and "facilitate" less.
Pacesetting	"Sets the pace". She/he sets high personal performance standards, leads by example and focuses on achieving results. If someone's performance is lagging, she/he will reassign the job to someone she/he considers more competent. Some team members may feel that this person needs to be more tolerant of other team members' views and working styles.

Table 14.1 (continued)

Authoritative	Provides a clear direction and takes the team forward with shared goals. She/he is particularly effective when a team or service has run into problems. The authoritative leader motivates team members by making it clear to them why what they do matters. She/he promotes commitment to the task and allows team members freedom to innovate.

affiliative, then democratic, then coaching. The pace-setting and coercive styles were associated with a negative impact, although it was acknowledged that all styles are useful in different contexts. The study showed that leaders who used a greater number of leadership styles, particularly those with a positive impact on organisational climate, performed better than those with a more limited repertoire. The most effective leaders switched between styles flexibly according to context. It was concluded that it was useful for individuals to be aware of their own style preferences so that they could expand their repertoire by developing their use of other styles.

The Goleman model of leadership styles has been applied to a range of professional groups, but there are few peer-reviewed published reports. Pennington [16] undertook a survey of principals of UK higher education colleges using both self- and third party- assessment. Principals of high-achieving colleges used more styles than principals of other colleges, and used their entire range more frequently. The principals at high achieving colleges were comparable to highly successful leaders in industry in terms of numbers of dominant and back-up styles, although used the democratic style more and the pace-setting style less frequently. This paper also concluded that self-perception about leadership style use was generally accurate. In the context of clinical leadership, an unpublished study of self-reported use of the six styles across senior NHS leaders, both clinical and managerial, concluded that the pace-setting style predominated, and that the coaching and commanding styles were least frequent [12, 19]. This conclusion appeared to support earlier work by Martin and Keogh [20] suggesting that the predominant leadership styles of physician managers were 'dominant' and 'conscientiousness,' where the former focused on control over tasks and the environment, directing others and achieving goals, while the latter related to independent working and a preference for working on tasks rather than dealing with people. The inference was that medical leaders needed to develop their 'people-oriented' rather than 'task oriented' leadership styles in order to move away from a transactional approach [21] towards a more effective transformational style of leadership [22, 23].

The second leadership style self-assessment tool used in this study was developed by Singh and Jampel [24], based on earlier work by Slevin and Pinto [25]. This model has been developed in the context of project management in the construction industry, and so has a more operational focus than Goleman's model. In the self-assessment tool that they describe, respondents are asked to answer 22 questions to determine the extent to which an individual leader invites information input from the team (I score) and involves the team in decision-making (D score). They defined five leadership styles, the most effective of which is the 'active manager,' that is, a leader who displays the most effective balance of consultative and independent decision-making activity (Table 14.2). They coined a new term for the visual readout of leadership style obtained through this approach: the leadership flexibility space. This 'space' is a box plot in which the individual leader's style is plotted based on consultative and independent decision-making propensity. The space is 'flexible' because although individual leaders can be placed anywhere within the space at a defined time point, they can move over time (for example with age or leadership training) or in varying contexts.

They applied this model to a group of engineers and found that the majority fell into the impoverished or consensus manager zones, with a very small number of active managers. There were no individuals in the consultative or complete autocrat zones, suggesting a negative, unhealthy culture in the organisation with limited

Table 14.2 Descriptions of leadership styles (adapted from [24])

Consultative autocrat	Takes information input from all but does not share decision-making. Decision-making may be efficient but may not fulfil the concerns shown by individual team members.
Complete autocrat	Neither takes anyone's input nor shares decision-making with anyone. Concerns shown by team members are not necessarily communicated to the leader or incorporated during the decision-making process. The leader sets his or her own agenda and expects others to follow.
Impoverished manager	Does not consult the group and will not make any decision by him/her self. All decisions are taken by the group in a random manner with no clear direction of travel. The leader is not aware of what is going on within the team. Chaos and disinterest can ensue.
Consensus manager	Involves the group in the whole decision-making process, letting the group decide by consensus. While this can be beneficial to team-building, the group may lack decisive leadership and a clear sense of direction. Decision-making may be very time-consuming.
Active manager	Able to make decisions independently, but will also share decision-making where appropriate. The leader consults the team and takes information input, is aware of the concerns of team members but also has a clear sense of the direction of travel of the team.

decision-making power, either due to intrinsic individual reluctance or to organisational restrictions. They concluded that the organisation should explore and correct cultural problems, and suggested a range of possible measures, including increasing delegation, leadership training and reviewing hiring and promotion criteria. In contrast to these results, however, another study in a similar setting found that the autocratic style dominated, with a smaller number of impoverished manager-style individuals [26].

Thus their model includes five distinct leadership styles, but these are based on only two underlying aspects of behaviour, and thus perhaps a more simplistic view of leadership styles than the Goleman model. However their description of its use in an engineering department does illustrate its practicality in terms of simplicity of administration and potential value to the organisation. This leadership style model may be most useful in exploring leadership in project management contexts, where there are short term projects with clear goals and timescales, rather than more complex leadership scenarios.

In the present study, the use of leadership styles by medical leaders was examined using an electronic SurveyMonkey® self-assessment questionnaire incorporating questions relating to each of the leadership style models outlined above. In the first part, respondents were asked to divide 100 percentage points across Goleman's six styles to self-assess their pattern of use of the styles in their leadership role. Percentage scores that respondents allocated to each of the six leadership styles were summated for the group. In the second section of the questionnaire, respondents answered 22 questions relating to the Singh and Jampel model. D and I scores for each individual were calculated and plotted on a grid, giving a visual read-out of the leadership style of each individual and of the group as a whole.

Two hundred and twenty four clinical and medical directors in hospital trusts across Yorkshire and Humber region (a large geographical region in England) were emailed with an explanation of the study and an electronic link to the questionnaire. There were responses from 78 of 224 clinical or medical directors (35%). 58/76 respondents who gave gender information were male (76%), and the median age group was 46–50 years. A wide range of clinical specialties was represented, the largest groups being medical, surgical, anaesthetics and diagnostics. 85% of respondents had had some previous leadership training: of these just under half (47%) had participated in a formal leadership course within their hospital, while 10% had undertaken an external course leading to an academic qualification.

Figure 14.1 shows the self-reported use of Goleman's six leadership styles across 78 respondents. The predominant styles reported overall were affiliative and democratic, with pace-setting the third most prevalent. Coaching and commanding styles were reported least frequently. There were no significant differences in reported leadership style use relating to gender, clinical specialty or whether or not the respondent worked in a foundation trust. Turning to the Singh and Jampel model, the majority of respondents mapped to the consensus manager style, that is, leaders who consult to a large extent but who show limited independent decision-making (Fig. 14.2). The active manager style was the second most frequent. A smaller number of individuals were consultative autocrats, that is, they consult but do not necessarily take the outcome of consultation into consideration when making decisions. The impoverished manager and complete autocrat styles were rarely seen.

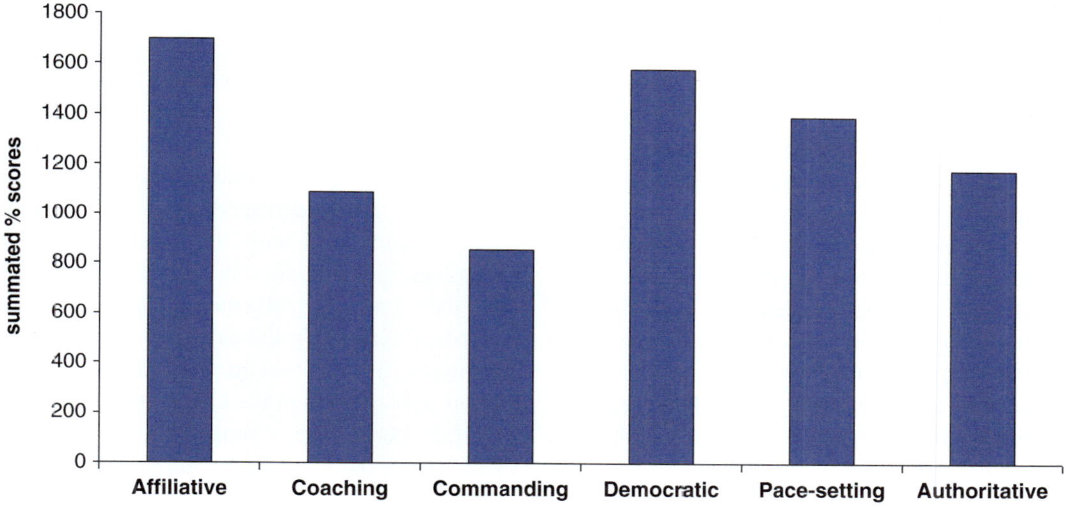

Fig. 14.1 Self-reported use of Goleman leadership styles (78 respondents)

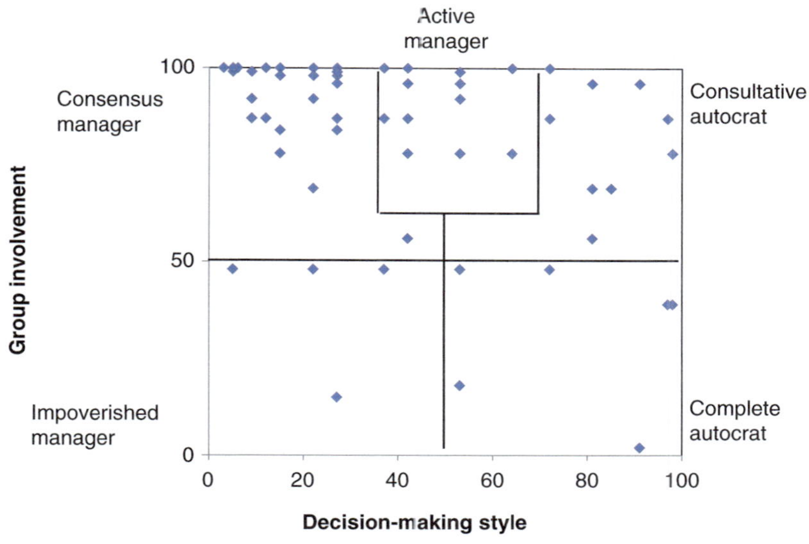

Fig. 14.2 Survey responses for Singh & Jampel leadership styles tool (n = 78)

In comparing the results using each of these self-assessment tools, it is clear that there are some areas of agreement. Firstly, both tools demonstrate that there is not a single 'typology' of medical leader, that is, not all leaders have the same pattern of use of leadership styles or behaviours. Furthermore both tools demonstrated a dominance of 'people-oriented' styles: in the Goleman model the affiliative and democratic styles were assessed across the group as being the most commonly used, while in the Singh and Jampel model, the most frequent styles were the consensus manager and the active manager. These results are in contrast to the previous perceptions of medical leaders as pace-setters and 'task oriented'.

There are a number of implications of this study. Individual leaders should critically explore (ideally using both self- and 360° assessment) their own use of leadership styles to determine which styles they use preferentially and which less frequently. Once the leader is aware of his/her style pattern, s/he can then consider how to increase the number of styles used routinely and the use of less preferred styles. This could be done either through reflective practice, or through targeted training, for example if a leader rarely uses the coaching style, then training in the principles of leading small group educational sessions could be useful.

At the organisational level knowledge of the leadership style preferences of individuals can aid the formation of effective teams combining people with a range of preferred styles. As an example, a team could be designed that includes an affiliative chief executive, who would foster links and a team spirit, with a pace-setting deputy who ensures that targets are met. Similarly, awareness of individuals' leadership styles at organisational level would be useful in allocating tasks, for example, the role of director of postgraduate education might be best suited to a leader with a predominant coaching style of leadership, while the head of service development would ideally have an authoritative style, with an ability to create and communicate a shared vision.

Finally, currently most leadership development programmes focus more on leadership skills than styles and it may be useful to incorporate learning and self-assessment relating to leadership style to provide learners with a more holistic approach to leadership development.

14.3 Study 2: Self-Assessment Using a Leadership Competency Framework

Health care organizations worldwide have sought to standardize and streamline the different skills required of leaders in healthcare. In the UK the NHS Institute for Innovation and Improvement undertook an intensive research program to develop an evidence-based competency framework. The Leadership Qualities Framework, first launched in 2002, identified a set of leadership qualities associated with the success of chief executives and directors in the health service. With the increasing realization of the importance of medical leadership in healthcare delivery, The Enhancing Engagement in Medical Leadership project was initiated in the UK in 2006 [27]. The Medical Leadership Competency Framework (MLCF), published in 2008, outlined the leadership competences required of doctors at various levels of seniority in order to help them to develop their skills to engage effectively in planning, provision and improvement of healthcare services [28–30]. It was increasingly recognized that in the complex healthcare environment organizational effectiveness depends on engagement of all team members and a shared sense of responsibility, and the MLCF promoted the concept of shared leadership, where leadership is not restricted to the people who hold a designated leadership role alone, but is part of the professional role of all doctors. The MLCF had five core domains: "Demonstrating Personal Qualities" (D1), "Working with others" (D2), "Managing Services" (D3), "Improving Services" (D4) and "Setting Direction" (D5), each of which is divided into four sub-domains. The framework was intended as a practical tool for personal development, and four competences are described for each sub-domain, with knowledge, skills and attitudes/behaviors outlined for each.

The MLCF was revised in the form of the Clinical Leadership Competency Framework [29] to broaden its applicability to other healthcare professional groups. In addition, the initial MLCF was updated to the NHS Leadership Framework [31] to extend its applicability to doctors at later stages in their careers. This new framework includes two additional domains: "Creating the Vision" (D6) and "Delivering the Strategy" (D7) (Fig. 14.3). More recently and in line with the changing and demanding context of the UK NHS, the NHS Leadership Academy has developed the Healthcare Leadership Model, which comprises a number of 'elements' organised into three broad categories relating to creating a sense of purpose, motivating individuals and teams, and improving system performance [32].

Competency frameworks have been criticised in that they focus too much on the individual leader instead of developing shared or distributed leadership which is considered an important drive to transform health care [33]. There has been a significant criticism of a 'leader-only' approach which overlooks important contextual influences that shape the focal construct of leadership at different levels [34, 35]. Leader-only approaches focus on "*the development of individual leaders through the enhancement of their personal attributes and qualities, behaviour and knowledge and skills - the creation of human capital*" [30, 36] whereas 'leadership development' is seen *as "a social influence process balancing order through the making and mending of relationships and is therefore a collective or shared activity, rather than an individual one*" [36]. There is however a need to develop leadership programmes based on the knowledge of the leaders to ensure that there is a direct fit between: the needs of the organisation; the aims of the programme and factors influencing motivation and or disengagement of participants with the programme. Competency frameworks have a part to play in developing self awareness of the leader's capability for 'leadership development' through initial 'leader development' as defined by Day [32]. This helps to focus on an individual leader's capacity to reliably self-determine their own leadership development needs in order to identify a level of individual readiness and preparedness to "*expand their capabilities in leadership roles and processes*" [34, 37, 38].

This study explored self-perception of UK Occupational Health Physicians (OHPs) on their leadership competency and training needs [39]. Participants in this study were members of the Society of Occupational Medicine (SOM) and Faculty of Occupational Medicine (FOM) of the

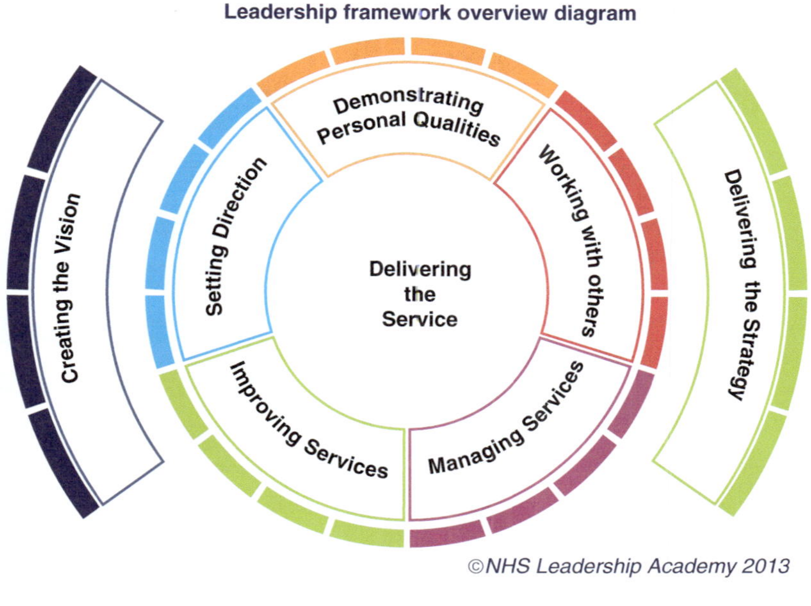

Fig. 14.3 NHS leadership framework

Royal College of Physicians who were working across a range of organisational contexts in including the statutory NHS, private healthcare, self-employed and in General Practice. They were sent a self-assessment e-questionnaire from the Society of Occupational Medicine (SOM) by email; a reminder email with the e-questionnaire followed two weeks later. Responses were returned to an email account and the data exported to an Excel spreadsheet.

The NHS England Leadership Academy Healthcare Leadership Framework [31] was used as a self-assessment leadership tool. In each domain of the Healthcare Leadership Framework, respondents were presented with eight leadership behaviours, two relating to each of the four sub-domains in that domain, and asked to rate their use of each behaviour as "a lot of the time," "some of the time" or "very little/none of the time." An individual who rated five or more of the eight behaviours in a domain as "all the time" was considered "confident" in that domain; otherwise s/he was considered "not confident." Mean leadership competency score under each domain was calculated by computing the total score of the group under the respective domain and dividing it by the number of responses.

Two hundred and fifty responses were received, representing 25% of the estimated study population. Whilst there are 1200 OHPs registered with the FOM, only approximately 1000 of them reside and work within the UK and were eligible to participate (personal communication). Of respondents, 66% were male, and the median age range was 51–60 years. 62% of had more than 15 years' experience in Occupational Medicine practice: 65% reported that they were self-employed or worked in the private sector, while 27% held an NHS post. Twenty eight percent reported that they had undertaken training in leadership and management leading to a degree or diploma while a further 45% had had brief training through their employing organisation.

The results of the study demonstrated that as a group, most OHPs (81.5%) had confidence in D1 (Demonstrating Personal Qualities). Approximately two-thirds (63.1%) of respondents were confident in D2 (Working with Others) followed by almost 57% in D3 (Managing Services). Only half (52.2%) had confidence in D4 (Improving Services). The numbers were however low when it came to D5 (Setting Direction—40.2%), D6 (Creating the Vision—26.5%) and D7 (Delivering the Strategy—34.5%) (Fig. 14.4). Looking at mean leadership competency scores for each of the domains similar results were obtained. Out of the maximum score of 8, the group scored 5.77 in D1 (Demonstrating Personal Qualities), followed by 5.16 in D2 (Working with Others), 4.62 in D3

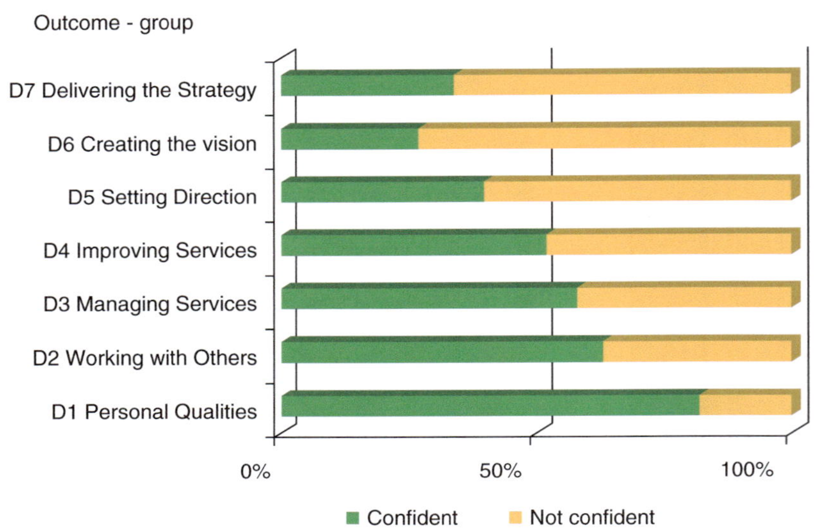

Fig. 14.4 Summated self-perception of competence confidence of respondents across the domains of the NHS leadership framework (n = 250)

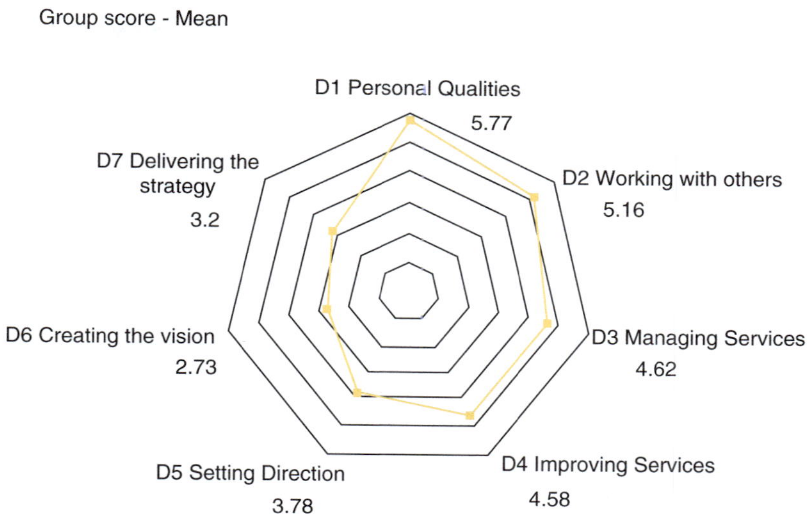

Fig. 14.5 Group leadership competency scores (n = 250)

(Managing Services) and 4.58 Improving Services (D4). The median score dropped below 50% level when it came to Setting Direction (D5, 3.78), Creating the Vision (D6, 2.73) or Delivering the Strategy (D7, 3.20) (Fig. 14.5).

Subgroup analysis demonstrated no differences between respondents relating to gender, age or years of experience as an OHP. Respondents who reported previous management experience had significantly higher confidence levels across all domains apart from D1 (Demonstrating Personal Qualities). Those with prior formal leadership and management training towards a diploma or degree had significantly higher confidence in D5 (Setting Direction) and D6 (Creating the vision). When questioned about their personal training needs, respondents as a group perceived a need for training across all the domains, but in particular domains 3–7: the domain where most reported a training need was domain 4 (Improving Services).

This self-assessment study has illustrated that doctors can self-assess their confidence across a range of leadership domains. The results demonstrate that OHPs in general lacked confidence in their leadership skills. OHPs were more confident in their personal qualities and team-working skills but struggled with the strategic aspects of leadership such as creating the vision and/or setting direction. Leadership and management experience had the most positive impact on OHPs' self-perceived competency level.

It is interesting to contrast these findings with those of Harris et al. [40] who explored self-assessment of leadership skills across doctors of three levels of seniority and across five sets of leadership skills. They found that early and mid level doctors had highest confidence in their decision-making, people management and communication skills, but lacked confidence in finance skills and strategic planning. Senior physician leaders displayed similar confidence levels across all five domains. Interestingly, mid level doctors who underwent leadership training demonstrated an increase in confidence across all domains but in particular financial management and communication skills, in agreement with this present study.

Most doctors, like OHPs, have a large clinical service delivery aspect to their professional role, involving many professional skills and attributes but in particular communication, time management, team-working and quality improvement/patient safety. Many doctors may lack confidence in setting direction, creating a vision or delivering a strategy, and may therefore choose not to engage in activities which require them to work within these domains. Targeted training to acquire the competences within these domains will empower them to develop their professional roles and take on new leadership challenges. This training could be acquired through attendance at courses or through self-directed study; some leadership models, for example the MLCF, have tools that can support personal development, and the appraisal process for career grade doctors, incorporating an annually updated personal development plan, is also useful in setting targets for development of leadership competences. However a further key requirement is support from colleagues: this may be informal through the leadership hierarchy of the organisation, or more formal coaching or mentoring [41].

Conclusions

While there is now broad acceptance that the degree of medical leadership and engagement in a healthcare organisation is directly related to the quality and productivity of that organisation, there is ambiguity as to how to support medical leadership development. It is not clear what is the optimal method of developing leadership skills and styles, nor the optimal balance of theoretical and practical learning, or taught versus self-directed learning. There is a need for further research to answer these questions, through evaluation of existing programmes and/or a broader exploration of the specific learning needs of individual or groups of leaders.

However, there is now a developing consensus that medical leadership development should to a greater or lesser extent be self-determined by medical leaders themselves [39, 42–44]. Both of the studies presented here demonstrate that it is possible to apply self-assessment to the field of medical leadership as a tool for personal development. These tools can be of value in targeting leadership development learning at an individual level. However such self-assessment tools cannot be used in isolation, and indeed have been accused of being reductionist [30]. There is a need for a deeper understanding of the place of self-assessment in the overall design and delivery of leadership development programmes, and as always, there is a need to share learning and good practice at a national (and international) level: nationally organisations that facilitate this include the International Academy of Medical Leadership, Faculty of Medical Leadership and Management and the NHS Leadership Academy.

One criticism of self-assessment in any field of competence is its reliability—although one study of leadership styles reported that self-assessment compared well with third party assessment [16], there is concern that self-assessment may not be accurate in determining learning needs [45], and furthermore that its accuracy may vary between individuals depending on their level of self-awareness [46]. Until we have definitive evidence that self-assessment is a valid method of determining learning needs, it would be wise to combine self-assessment with other assessment methods to ensure that the development needs of individuals have been accurately determined and are being met.

In conclusion, we have much to learn about how best to develop leadership skills and behaviours in medical leaders now and in the future. However the clear association between medical leadership and organisational effectiveness suggests that this is an area where the greater understanding will yield greater improvements in quality and cost-effectiveness of healthcare.

References

1. Ham C. Improving the performance of health services: the role of clinical leadership. Lancet. 2003;361:1978–80.
2. Kumar RDC. Leadership in healthcare. Anaesth Intensiv Care Med. 2013;14:39–41.
3. Eckert R, West M, Altman D, Steward K, Pasmore B. Delivering a collective leadership strategy for health care. London: Centre for Creative Leadership: The Kings Fund; 2014.
4. Shipton H, Armstrong C, West M, Dawson J. The impact of leadership and quality climate on hospital performance. Int J Qual Health Care. 2008;20(6):439–45.
5. Smith E. Review of centrally funded improvement and leadership development functions. London: NHS; 2015.

6. West M, Eckert R, Steward K, Pasmore B. Developing collective leadership for health care. London: The Centre for Creative Leadership: The Kings Fund; 2014.
7. Francis Robert QC. Report of the Mid Staffordshire NHS Foundation Trust Public Inquiry. [Online]. Last accessed 20 November 2016 at: http://www.midstaffspublicinquiry.com/report. 2013.
8. Kennedy I. The Report of the public enquiry into children's heart surgery at Bristol Royal Infirmary 1984–1995; learning from Bristol. London: Department of Health; 2001.
9. Keogh B. Review into the quality of treatment provided by 14 hospital trusts in England: overview report. London: Department of Health; 2013.
10. Darzi A. High quality care for all: NHS next stage review final report. London: Department of Health. [Online]. Last accessed 20 November 2016 at: http://www.official-documents.gov.uk/document/cm74/7432/7432.pdf. 2008.
11. Stoll L, Swanwick T, Foster-Turner J, Moss F. Leadership development for junior doctors: what can we learn from 'Darzi' fellowships in clinical leadership? Int J Leadersh Public Serv. 2011;7:273–86.
12. The King's Fund. Leadership and engagement for improvement in the NHS: together we can. London: The King's Fund; 2012.
13. Frich C, Brewster AL, Cherlin EJ, Bradley EH. Leadership development programmes for physicians: a full systematic literature review. J Gen Int Med. 2015;30(5):656–74.
14. Ham C, Clark J, Spurgeon P, Dickinson H, Armit K. Doctors who became chief executives in the NHS: from keen amateurs to skilled professionals. J R Soc Med. 2011;104:113–9.
15. Kung JW, Slanetz PJ, Huang GC, Eisenberg RL. Reflective practice: assessing its effectiveness to teach professionalism in a radiology residency. Acad Radiol. 2015;22:1280–6.
16. Pennington J. Further lessons in leadership. Manag Educ. 2003;17:24–8.
17. Chapman ALN, Johnson D, Kilner K. Leadership styles used by senior medical leaders: patterns, influences and implications for leadership development. Leadersh Health Serv. 2014;27(4):283–98.
18. Goleman D. Leadership that gets results. Harvard business review. March–April 2000. Boston, MA: Harvard Business School; 2000.
19. Santry C. Resilient NHS managers lack required leadership skills, DH research says. Health Service Journal, 6 July. [online] Last accessed 20 November 2016 at: www.hsj.co.uk/news/workforce/resilient-nhs-managers-lack-required-leadership-skills-dh-researchsays/5032248.article. 2011.
20. Martin WF, Keogh TJ. Managing medical groups: 21st century challenges and the impact of physician leadership styles. J Med Pract Manage. 2004;20:102–6.
21. Schwartz RW, Tumblin TF. The power of servant leadership to transform health care organizations for the 21st-century economy. Arch Surg. 2002;137:1419–27.
22. Mccue JD, Magrinat G, Hansen CJ, Bailey RS. Residents' leadership styles and effectiveness as perceived by nurses. J Med Educ. 1986;61:53–8.
23. Xiragasar S, Samuels ME, Stoskopf CH. Physician leadership styles and effectiveness: an empirical study. Med Care Res Rev. 2005;62:720–40.
24. Singh A, Jampel G. Leadership flexibility space. J Manag Eng. 2010;26:176–87.
25. Slevin DP, Pinto JK. Project leadership: understanding and consciously choosing your style. Proj Manag J. 1991;22:39–47.
26. Oke AE, Gbadura IH. An examination of project management leadership styles of Nigerian quantity surveyors. J Build Perform. 2010;1:57–63.
27. Medical Leadership Competency Framework. Coventry: NHS institute for innovation and improvement. [Online]. Last accessed 20 November 2016 at: http://www.leadershipacademy.nhs.uk/wp-content/uploads/2012/11/NHSLeadership-Leadership-Framework-Medical-Leadership-Competency-Framework-3rd-ed.pdf. 2010.
28. Spurgeon P, Mazelan PM, Barwell F. Medical engagement: a crucial underpinning to organizational performance. Health Serv Manag Res. 2011;24(3):114–20.
29. Clinical Leadership Competency Framework. Coventry: NHS Institute for Innovation and Improvement. [Online]. Last accessed 20 November 2016 at: http://www.leadershipacademy.nhs.uk/wp-content/uploads/2012/11/NHSLeadership-Leadership-Framework-Clinical-Leadership--Competency-Framework-CLCF.pdf. 2011.
30. Edmonstone J. Whither the elephant?: the continuing development of clinical leadership in the UK national health services. Int J Plann Manag. 2014;29:280–91.
31. The Leadership Framework. Coventry: NHS Institute for Innovation and Improvement. [Online]. Last accessed 20 November 2016 at: www.leadershipacademy.nhs.uk/develop-your-leadership-skills/leadership-framework/the-framework-overview. 2011.
32. Storey J, Holti R. Towards a new model of leadership for the NHS. NHS Leadership Academy. [Online]. Last accessed 20 November 2016 at: http://www.leadershipacademy.nhs.uk/wp-content/uploads/2013/05/Towards-a-New-Model-of-Leadership-2013.pdf. 2013.
33. West M, Armit K, Loewenthal L, Eckert R, West T, Lee A. Leadership and leadership development in health care: the evidence base. London: Faculty of Medical Leadership and Management; 2015.
34. Day DV. Leadership development: a review in context. Leadersh Q. 2000;11:581–613.
35. Day DV, Harrison MM. Multilevel, identity-based approach to leadership development. Hum Resour Manag Rev. 2007;17:360–73.

36. Edmonstone J. Developing leaders and leadership in healthcare: a case for rebalancing? Leadersh Health Serv. 2011;24(1):8–18.
37. Van Velsor E, McCauley CD. Our view of leadership development. In: McCauley CD, Van Velsor E, editors. The centre for creative leadership handbook of leadership development. San Francisco: Jossey Bass; 2004. p. 1–22.
38. Solansky ST. Self determination and leader development. Manag Learn. 2015;46(5):618–35.
39. Giri P, Aylott J, Kilner K. Self-determining medical leadership needs of occupational health physicians: leadership in health services (paper in press). 2017.
40. Harris MB, von Keudell A, McMahon G, Bierer B. Physician self-assessment of leadership skills. Physician Exec. 2014;40(2):30–4.
41. Mckenna MK, Gartland MP, Pugno PA. Development of physician leadership competencies: perceptions of physician leaders, physician educators and medical students. J Health Adm Educ. 2004;21(3):343–54.
42. Aylott J, Kilner K, Breen B, Chapman ALN, Giri P, Withers M, WIN T. Participation and engagement by design: maximising the return on investment of medical and clinical leadership and quality improvement projects. In: Presentation at The 7th International Conference for Evidence Based Healthcare Teachers ad Developers: Evidence for Sustainability of healthcare, increasing value, reducing waste, Taormina (Italy) 28–31 October, 2015.
43. Nassef A. Medical leadership and systems transformation: paper presented to the centre for leadership annual conference. Sheffield: Sheffield Hallam University; 2016.
44. Nassef A, Aylott J. Doctors in Co-design of a medical leadership programme: self-determination at sheffield teaching hospitals NHS trust, UK. In: Paper presented at The 6th International Conference on Self-Determination Theory, Victoria, BC; 2016
45. Dunning D, Heath C, Suls JM. Flawed self assessment: implications for health, education and the workplace. Psychol Sci Public Interest. 2004;5(3):69–106.
46. Atwater LE, Yammarino FJ. Does self-other agreement on leadership perceptions moderate the validity of leadership and performance predictions? Pers Psychol. 1992;45:141–64.

15 Strategic Management

Branko Perunovic, Louise Dunk, and Jill Aylott

We can't keep up with the pace of change, let alone get ahead of it… The hierarchical structures and organizational processes we have used for decades to run and improve our enterprises are no longer up to the task of winning in this faster-moving world.

John Kotter [1]

Beyond doubt, the healthcare sector and the majority of organisations within it are at the strategic inflection point. This concept, first introduced by Andy Grove, the former CEO of Intel, argues that in the life cycle of any organisation and industry inevitably comes a time when the 'rules of the game' change fast and forever. The circumstances invariably change in such a radical way that its participants have to change the way they do things if they wish to prosper in a new environment, but if they fail to adapt, they risk extinction [2]. The scope and speed of political, economic, societal and technological changes and the environmental landscape affect all sectors of society, including healthcare. The scope and speed of changes political, economic, societal, technological and environmental landscape is affecting all sectors of society, including healthcare [3, 4]. In the healthcare industry it manifests as a mismatch between demand and human and capital resources available [5–7].

In the UK, the new National Health Service (NHS) milieu is outlined in Five Year Forward View [8] and the subsequent framework for implementation as Sustainability and Transformation Plans (STP) [9]. General themes are as expected and follow the World Health Organisations views on global health care transformation, with health services moving from fragmentation to integration, consolidation, convergence and connectivity in order to achieve better health outcomes for the population, whilst a global demand to reduce costs and increase efficiency to demonstrate value, will intensify [10, 11]. Not surprisingly, there is a lot of emphasis on general practice, maintenance of health and wellbeing, targeted early intervention in home and community and more services provided in non-hospital settings either through primary care or by new integrated providers. As expected, there are no easy answers, neither now nor in the prospect, on where the funding and time for transformation will come from, how the continuous engagement of the frontline clinical and community teams, carers and patients are going to be embedded in the journey. Also, it is not clear if and when the permissive legislative interventions will be put in place to relieve tensions between organisation-based statutory framework and emerging place-based model to enable more effective coordination of activity across the exist-

B. Perunovic (✉) • L. Dunk
Sheffield Teaching Hospitals NHS Foundation Trust, Sheffield, UK
e-mail: Branko.Perunovic@sth.nhs.uk; Louise.Dunk@wales.nhs.uk

J. Aylott
Directorate for International MBA Programmes, International Academy of Medical Leadership, Sheffield, UK
e-mail: Jill.Aylott@iamedicalleadership.com

P. Godbole et al. (eds.), *Why Hospitals Fail*, DOI 10.1007/978-3-319-56224-7_15

ing organisational boundaries [12]. Although there are substantial contextual differences, the magnitude of challenge in the UK does not differ from those found elsewhere in the developed and developing world. Key drivers shaping new global healthcare milieu- austerity and rising demand—are ubiquitous. They are synergistically creating the environment dominated by volatility, uncertainty, complexity and ambiguity [13]. Where once there were reasonably simple choices and apparent predictability, choices and consequences are less clear and the outdated strategic management methods do not instil much hope.

Strategy is often considered to be the pinnacle of managerial activity. The word "strategy" is overused and it is often very difficult to distil the essence of strategy from the motivational speak that is supposed to stimulate organisational efforts towards proclaimed goals or 'big picture' jargon that is often oblivious to the plethora of local contexts. Also, it is often seen as detached from explicit actions required for implementation of interventions required for safeguarding the prosperity of the organisation, its patients, other users and partners.

Strategy needs to be seen as "a cohesive and coherent response to an important challenge" [14]. The painful truth about strategy is that we need it only because the resources are finite—in the utopian world with unlimited resources we would not need one. Therefore, a good strategy is largely about identifying critical issues and focusing resources to address them.

In all healthcare ecosystems, there is an unavoidable tension between the short term focus on operational and financial targets and medium to long term focus on the quality of care. Although no one can or should be oblivious to the finances or unwarranted operational variations [15], it is becoming obvious that healthcare organisations should not be discouraged from pursuing alternatives that create long term value through the focus on the patients' and carers' needs through "sustained and comprehensive commitment to quality improvement" [11]. In most healthcare systems, the NHS not being an exception, there is also "an ideological rift between advocates of central control and supporters of devolution" [16], the latter advocating clinician-led quality agenda [17, 18] and devotion to "continual learning and improvement of patient care, top to bottom and end to end" [19].

A recent UK survey showed that there may be a gap in the management education [20]. This is especially evident in the cohort of senior medical managers, most of whom did not have an opportunity to have a structured management training. The UK survey supports global findings that there is a "capability gap" in healthcare which is likely to present talent-related challenges over the coming years. The ten human resource challenges include: culture and engagement; leadership; learning and development, reinventing HR; workforce on demand; performance management; HR and people analytics; simplification of work; machines as talent and big data everywhere. The "capability gap" appears to be increasing in magnitude year on year as the accelerating economy and rapid changes in the workforce have created even more urgency [10, 21]. The traditional models of workforce development in management and leadership will need to be 'disrupted' to rise to the challenges ahead for medical and non-medical managers alike, will need to re-think fundamental concepts of strategic management and practice them within a value-based-healthcare framework [22, 23], passionately focusing on pursuing quality, adaptability and resilience. There is a global move towards a transition to outcome or Value Based Care (VBC) payment models, which seek to align costs with quality and outcome measures[10]. The bottom line is that, the healthcare organisations of the future will have to learn to constantly reinvent themselves, and transform through improvement and innovation in a timely and purposeful manner [24].

Having that in mind, we did not design this chapter as a 'strategic management manual'. Our goal was to draw your attention to some basic concepts and encourage you the reader to explore this topic further by referring you authors such as Mintzberg [25, 26], Porter [27, 28], Christensen

[29], Govindarajan [30], McGrath [31] and Kotter [32, 33].

15.1 Between Deliberate and Emerging Strategies

The concepts of formal *planning*, aimed at enabling companies to develop the best fit between themselves and the environment, emerged in the business community in 1920s with the introduction of the Harvard Policy Model.[1] After the Second World War, a group of former military planners, engaged to address Ford Motor Company's growing financial and administrative problems, successfully introduced financial and procedural discipline and advanced concepts of *strategic planning* to this corporation and later to the world of mainstream business and government. Although this was more or less an annual budgeting exercise, the concept of *strategic planning* worked well in the following two decades. However, in the 1970s, Japanese companies and a fluctuation of oil prices started to mount a challenge. The new approach, *strategic management,* was about connecting the planning process to the 'real world' where strategy is played out through seamless amalgamation of strategic planning and operational management [34].

The individual organisation's style of strategic management sits somewhere on the continuum between, so called, *deliberate* and *emerging* strategy models [35]. Formulation of *deliberate strategies* is a top-down process and is seen as pre-requisite of the 'central leadership'. Once it is done, it is passed to other members of the organisation for implementation. Since entrusted with large funds and mandate to realise a defined set of operational and financial outcomes, large organisations and governmental institutions are largely inclined towards a deliberate, top-down approach. However, there are inherent fallacies associated with planning of any kind [25]. First is the fallacy of *predetermination*—one may erroneously believe that it is possible to 'know the future' and prepare for the exact set of events. That does not mean that one should not plan, but one needs "… to plan the way a fire department plans: it cannot anticipate where the next fire will be, so it has to shape an energetic and efficient team that is capable of responding to the unanticipated as well as ordinary event" [2]. The second fallacy is that of *detachment*. In large or bureaucratic organisations, those who formulate strategy are often removed from implementation and a direct operational contact with the environment. Rich and true data that aggregate into strategically meaningful intelligence rest with those who deal with the patients/service users and the service users themselves. Middle managers and frontline staff are also those that are first to spot that what worked before is not working any more. An inclusive approach to strategic management may provide a critical advantage in the volatile environment. And finally, the fallacy of *formalisation* refers to common beliefs that innovation and competitive advantage can be generated only by analysis and structure, without active experimentation. This can only lead to 'petrification' of strategy and inertia to integrate, synthesize, or create options for new directions.

At the other end of strategic continuum is *the emerging approach.* Humans think in order to act, but also act in order to think and organisations are learning what works in practice. 'Experiments' that work should converge gradually into viable strategies as intentions collide with and accommodate a changing reality. Today, these ideas may have more appeal as we are looking for strategic flexibility in all segments of society, including healthcare.

15.2 Seven Step Strategic Management Process and Strategy Review

However, even if a balance of the common approach to strategic management on the deliberate-emerging continuum tends to tilt towards the *deliberate approach*, and the formal annual planning routines and rituals

[1]The structured assessment of Strengths, Weaknesses, Opportunities, and Threats (SWOT) came from this school.

remain business-as-usual; this balance needs to be set and monitored intentionally and intelligently through a frequent and routine *strategy review* process. It requires a conscious effort, focus, practice and willingness of organisation to constantly reinvent itself and, when required, to pivot, sometimes painfully, but always in a timely manner and with the constancy of purpose. This is all challenging because when under pressure, organisations become inward oriented and its members tend to become risk-averse creatures-of-habit rather than innovative and enterpreneurial.

We recommend a continuous, seven–step strategic management framework, which, as we said, incorporates a deliberate, frequent and routine strategy review process aimed to health-check the whole seven-step sequence. This approach should keep the organisational strategy relevant and context sensitive and enable organisations to remain sensitive to changes in the environment and change in a timely and purposeful manner if and when required.

15.2.1 Articulating the Strategic Intent and Defining the Mission

The foundation for strategic management is laid by the hierarchy of strategic intent [36]. The strategic intent articulates the long term intention of the organisation, its unique point of view about the future, provides the sense of direction and focuses the emotional and intellectual energy required for acquiring capabilities and resources to make the desired future possible. It must not be misguided, vague or without a focus [14]. Strategic intent is expressed through organisation's vision and mission statements. A vision statement communicates organisation's desired future position to its members. A mission statement, on the other hand, relates an organization to the society and provides its stakeholders and members with the framework and purpose. A purposeful mission statement needs to answer four questions: What does the organisation do? How does it do it? Whom does it do it for? What value is it bringing?

It is very important for every organisation to frequently reflect on its strategic intent and monitor the gap between its resources and ambitions and, when necessary, regenerate its strategic core.

15.2.2 Exploring and Refining a Business Models

A business model defines the organisation's structure and its methods for generating revenues. An organisation may need to have a number of business models for different units or aspects of its operations, but it is vital that they are all guided by the strategic intent and act synergistically. Business modelling and its constant refinement is an important part of the strategic process, because without a viable business model foundations of an organisation would be built on shaky ground.

Every business model can be broken down to nine building blocks: customer segments, value proposition, customer relationships, channels, revenue stream, key activities, key partners, key resources and cost structure [37]. A consistency in applying this approach is helpful to understand the web of functional co-dependencies and constraints across the supply and demand chains, as well as human, financial and material resources required to offer the best possible service to patients now and in the future.

15.2.3 Setting Goals and Objectives

Whilst the strategic intention, mission and business models explain the organisation's philosophy, goals and objectives define the end results to be achieved. Goals are often seen as broad categories and the objectives represent end outcomes of accomplished goals. Objectives may be set for any organisational domain to benchmark clinical, financial, HR or operational performance. They can also serve as a motivating agent, an instrument for making decisions or to define the relationship with the environment. Objectives are multiple and need to be set to reflect the balance of organisational variables and the reality of external and internal constraints. They must be set to be challenging, but attainable, understandable, concrete and with specific timeframes. In the complex healthcare environment, many organisational objectives are set externally and remotely.

15.2.4 Understanding the Environment

Understanding and adapting to changes in the environment is fundamental for the organisational survival. It is practical to think of the environment as a set of three concentric layers: macro-environment, industry/sector and competitors/markets. Each of them provides different levels of granularity. Systematic scanning of the environment and analysing information to generate useful business intelligence needs to be seen as a continuous activity that feeds to the other steps of the strategic process. Gathering and sharing information and assembling it into useful intelligence need to be a continuous responsibility of all members of an organisation, with the particular emphasis, on those who are regularly in a direct contact with patients/service users and other organisations or agencies.

There are a number of methods to assist with analysis of the environment and they are part of every contemporary textbook [38] or a management manual [39]. Most are simple to learn, but take time and effort to practice candidly, inclusively and consistently.

Useful tools for assessing macro-environment are *PESTLE* and *scenario analysis*. *PESTLE* is mnemonic which stands for Political, Economic, Societal, Technological, Legal and Environmental. The aim of this method is to give a bird's eye view, consistently check all six domains and identify key drivers for change. *Scenario analysis* has been developed as a method for analysing outcomes of strategic approaches to alternative futures and this method proved its worth for assessing volatile and complex environments [40, 41].

Effects of macro-environmental factors surface within groups of organisations that provide essentially the same services—within the industry/sector layer. *Porter's Five Forces analysis* is a useful tool for understanding the structure and attractiveness of an industry by analysing the interplay of 'five forces' that shape competition. These are: extent of rivalry between competitors, power of buyers, power of suppliers, threat of substitutes and threat of new entrants [42].

To understand the layer below the industry—competitors and markets- one should focus on analysis of *strategic groups* and *market segments*. *Strategic groups* represent cohorts of organisations within an industry with similar strategic characteristics. They may be deploying similar strategies or models for competition. Strategic group analysis is essential to understand direct competition, map strategic opportunities and assess barriers for exploiting these opportunities or even for moving the activity to new market spaces where the competition is minimised [43]. *Market segments* represent groups of customers who have similar needs that are distinct from the needs of customers in other parts of the market. A *"niche"* is a colloquialism for a small market segment. Analysis of market segments provides insights about variation of customer needs and enables building of secure segmentation strategy by focusing on those needs that are highly distinctive from those typical in the other parts of the market.

In a volatile environment, it is also important to look into 'areas' which are not necessarily adequately captured through analysis of industry, competitors or markets. Rita McGrath developed a term "arena", to describe connection between market segment, offer and geographic location, characterised by particular "connections between customers and solutions, not by conventional offering that are more or less substitutes for one another" [31].

15.2.5 Formulation of Strategy

This stage is about taking decisions on what to do to get from where one is to where one wants to be. As importantly, at this stage one needs to decide what not to do. As Richard Rumelt emphasised: "a strategy does not remove scarcity and its consequence – the necessity of choice… Not miscalculation, bad strategy is avoidance of the hard work of crafting good strategy. One common reason for choosing avoidance is the pain or difficulty of choice" [14].

The core of good strategy comprises three elements: a *diagnosis* that explains the challenge, *a guiding policy* as an general approach for dealing with challenge and set of *coherent actions* that are designed to carry out the guiding policy [14]. In many organisations the process stops with the formulation of a guiding policy—but a guiding policy is not a synonym for strategy. On the contrary, strategy is about actions, about a set of coherent and coordinated actions which build upon each other and focus organisational energy towards the chosen goals. A coherence and coordination need to be introduced to the system by design but, in keeping with the pace of change in today's world, this will also need a constant adjustment in line with the emergent reality, and protection from being hijacked by 'mutual adjustments' or compromises to accommodate ad-hoc interests of various stakeholders.

15.2.6 Implementation of Strategy

Carrying out actions for implementing strategy is where the rubber meets the road. From the management perspective this is an active process with leaders at all levels being actively involved in supervision and refinement of actions. This includes a proactive 'engineering' of the organisational culture, not just top-down setting of targets and delegating. An approach best suited for the challenges of today needs to focus on distributed leadership, flexibility, adaptability and development of organisational capabilities and behaviours required to sustain the transition [44]. It is epitomised by the concept of learning organisations [45] and discussed further in Chap. 13. Learning organisations support experimentation, and have a healthy attitude towards risk and failure. They have low inertia, both when embarking on the journey and when changing directions. A learning organisation does not have a disconnect between the strategy and its execution, and has developed capabilities to avoid a number of common 'pathologies of execution'. First, there is no omission of responsibility—everyone has a good idea of the decisions and actions in own remit. Second, there is no overreach—the capabilities and resources are constantly been developed in such a way to match the task. Finally, the information flows free throughout the organisation—implementation of strategy relies on good communication and sharing up-to-date intelligence, so all members of the organisation are enabled to understand impacts of their choices.

15.2.7 Control

Finally, in order to see through the implementation of strategy to successful completion, organisations need to create effective control mechanisms. Strategic control differs from other forms of management control. It is focused on realization of *future goals* and must be able to deal with complexity, ambiguity and uncertainty at all steps of the strategic management process. The effective strategic management requires four types of control mechanisms, all of which exist to alert to emerging 'gaps' between the intentions and reality and address them effectively. *Implementation Control* follows implementation both in terms of individual steps and the whole strategy. *Special Alert Control* is to enable rigorous and timely reassessment of organisational strategy should unforeseen significant events occur. *Premise Control* is designed to check systematically and constantly if the premises or predictions on which a strategy is based are still valid. *Strategic Surveillance* is designed to track a range of relevant sources within and outside of the organisation and identify issues or events that may have impact on the organisational strategy [46].

Strategic management is one of the most complex acts of any organisation. Well designed and implemented, it may prove to make all the difference between prosperity and struggle for hospitals facing the strategic inflection point brought by profound societal, technological and economic changes. For many organisations successful strategic management process will require a shift along three interconnected perspectives.

First, hospitals will need to design and put in place strategic management processes fit for purpose. For example, a comprehensive and continuous seven step process will enable hospitals to deeply root themselves in the environment in which they provide service, and align their strategy, operations, resources and culture. Second, hospitals will need to invest resources to service this function. The main one is dedicated time of their medical and non-medical managers, and there is no shortcut here. Without frequent reflection and refocusing, managers inevitably default to a 'maintenance engineer' mindset—chasing targets or 'rightsizing'—rather than being agents of change through building competences and resources required for the future. Therefore, strategy reviews must not become a synonym or sidelined by performance or financial reviews—these are all important, but different organisational functions. And finally, the strategic management needs to be an inclusive, engaging and holistic function of the organisation, not a set of loosely connected niche conversations within the organisational structure, individual units or professional groups. To be effective in the emerging healthcare milieu, the process will also have to span across the organisational boundaries and engage all stakeholders, staying particularly attuned to the voices of the primary service users- patients and their families.

References

1. Kotter JP. Accelerate! Harv Bus Rev. 2012;90:44–58.
2. Grove AS. Only the paranoid survive: how to exploit the crisis points that challenge every company and career. London: HarperCollins; 1997, c1996.
3. Schwab K. The fourth industrial revolution. Cologny: World Economic Forum; 2016.
4. Winston AS. The big pivot : radically practical strategies for a hotter, scarcer, and more open world. Boston: Harvard Business Review Press; 2014.
5. CGI. Healthcare challenges and trends: the patient at the heart of care. CGI; 2014.
6. Deloitte. UK healthcare and life sciences predictions2020. Johannesburg: Deloitte; 2014.
7. World Health Organisation. Health systems financing. The path to universal coverage. Geneva: World Health Organisation; 2010.
8. NHS England. Five year forward view. England: NHS; 2014.
9. NHS England. Delivering the forward view: NHS planning guidance 2016/17 – 2020/21. England: NHS; 2016.
10. Deloitte. 2016 Global health care outlook. Battling costs while improving care. Johannesburg: Deloitte; 2016.
11. Ham C, Berwick DM, Dixon J. Improving quality in the English NHS A strategy for action. London: Kings Fund; 2016.
12. Alderwick H, Dunn MC, Mckenna K, Walsh N, Ham C. Sustainability and transformation plans in the NHS. How are they being developed in practice? London: Kings Fund; 2016.
13. Deloitte. Fit4VUCA. Towards a risk intelligent culture. Johannesburg: Deloitte; 2014.
14. Rumelt RP. Good strategy/bad strategy: the difference and why it matters. London: Profile; 2011.
15. Lord Carter of Coles. Operational productivity and performance in English NHS acute hospitals: unwarranted variation. Department of Health; 2016.
16. Leatherman S, Sutherland K. The quest for quality: refining the NHS reforms a policy analysis and chartbook. London: Nuffield Trust; 2008.
17. Department of Health. High quality care for all: NHS next stage review final report. Department of Health; 2008.
18. Stoller JK, Goodall A, Baker A. Why the best hospitals are managed by doctors. 2016. Available from: https://hbr.org/2016/12/why-the-best-hospitals-are--managed-by-doctors [Accessed 29 Dec 2016].
19. National Advisory Group on the Safety of Patients in England. A promise to learn – a commitment to act: improving the safety of patients in England. London: Department of Health; 2013.
20. Powell A, Davies H. Managing doctors, doctors managing. Marylebone: Nuffield Trust; 2016.
21. Deloitte. Global human capital trends 2016 the new organization: different by design. Johannesburg: Deloitte; 2015.
22. Alderwick H, Robertson R, Appleby J, Dunn P, Maguire D. Better value in the NHS. The role of changes in clinical practice. London: Kings Fund; 2015.
23. Porter ME, Lee TH. The strategy that will fix health care. Harv Bus Rev. 2013;91:50–70.

24. Nunes P, Breene T. Reinvent your business before it's too late. Harv Bus Rev. 2011;89(1/2):80–7.
25. Mintzberg H. The rise and fall of strategic planning. Harlow: Financial Times Prentice Hall; 2000.
26. Mintzberg H. Tracking strategies : toward a general theory. Oxford: Oxford University Press; 2007.
27. Magretta J. Understanding Michael Porter : the essential guide to competition and strategy. Boston: Harvard Business Review Press; 2012. c2012
28. Porter ME. Competitive advantage: creating and sustaining superior performance. New York: Free Press; 1998.
29. Christensen CM. The innovator's dilemma. New York: HarperBusiness; 2000.
30. Govindarajan V. Ten rules for strategic innovators : from idea to execution. Boston: Harvard Business School Press; 2005. c2005
31. Mcgrath RGA. The end of competitive advantage: how to keep your strategy moving as fast as your business foreword by Alex Gourlay, Alliance Boots. Boston: Harvard Business Review Press; 2013. [2013]
32. Kotter JP. Leading change. Boston: Harvard Business School Press; 1996. c1996
33. Kotter JP. Accelerate : building strategic agility for a faster moving world/John P. Kotter. Boston: Harvard Business Review Press; 2014. [2014]
34. Gluck FW, Kaufman SF, Walleck AS, Mcleod K, Stuckey J. Thinking strategically. McKinsey Quarterly; 2000.
35. Mintzberg H, Waters JA. Of strategies, deliberate and emergent. Strateg Manag J. 1985;6:257–72.
36. Hamel G, Prahalad CK. Strategic Intent. Harv Bus Rev. 1989;67:63–78.
37. Osterwalder A. Business model generation : a handbook for visionaries, game changers, and challengers. Hoboken: John Wiley; 2010.
38. Johnson G. Exploring strategy. Harlow: Pearson; 2014.
39. Berg GVDA. Key management models: the 75+ models every manager needs to know/Gerben van den Berg, Paul Pietersma. Harlow: Pearson Education Limited; 2015.
40. Schwartz P. The art of the long view New York. New York: Doubleday/Currency; 1991. c1991
41. Van Der Heijden K. Scenarios: the art of strategic conversation. Chichester: Wiley; 2005.
42. Porter ME. The five competitive forces that shape strategy. Harv Bus Rev. 2008;86:78–93.
43. Kim WC. Blue ocean strategy : how to create uncontested market space and make the competition irrelevant. Boston: Harvard Business Review Press; 2015.
44. Best A, Greenhalgh T, Lewis S, Saul JE, Carroll S, Bitz J. Large-system transformation in health care: a realist review. Milbank Q. 2012;90:421–56.
45. Senge PM. The fifth discipline: the art and practice of the learning organization, Century Business; 1992.
46. Ruefli T, Sarrazin J. Strategic control of corporate development under ambiguous circumstances. Manag Sci. 1981;27:1158–70.

16 Transformation, Efficiency and Effectiveness in Hospitals

Prasad Godbole

16.1 Introduction

We have already seen in the introductory chapter that a 'successful' hospital relies on the fine balance between performance (the activity delivered) along with the finance and patient safety (quality and effectiveness). Where patient safety or quality fails; more finance is required to correct the problem leaving less finance to maintain performance targets. Where less finances are provided to deliver a certain amount of activity, corners may be cut to save money and have an adverse impact on patient safety and quality.

Globally there is an increasing need for hospitals to save money, keep patients safe but at the same time delivering cutting edge treatments to patients consistently [1]. Furthermore increasing competition between hospitals to provide timely healthcare services has led to a sharp focus on strategies that look at all three elements that make a 'successful' hospital.

This chapter will explore the commonly used terms of transformation, efficiency and effectiveness in hospital healthcare delivery and should be read in conjunction with the introductory chapter and the chapters on leadership and change. Case studies and examples are provided to illustrate the salient points. Efficiency and effectiveness will be discussed first and secondly we will explore how both will impact on the transformation of healthcare.

16.2 Efficiency

Let us look at a scenario. If a surgeon can do five operations on a 4 hour operating schedule and each operation generates an income of $2000 (total $10,000). Assume the costs of running the operating room for the 4 hours is $3000. This leaves the organisation with a gross profit of $7000. Now if another surgeon can do six similar operations in the same time with the same outcomes then the costs of running the operating room remain the same but the total gross profit increases to $9000. If you are the Executive Director responsible for the operating rooms which would you prefer? Obviously the second surgeon as he can do more for the same cost. This means that the second surgeon is deemed to be more efficient than the first. **Efficiency** is the (often measurable) ability to avoid wasting materials, energy, efforts, money, and time in doing something or in producing a desired result. In a more general sense, it is the ability to do things well, successfully, and without waste. In simple terms in hospitals it means doing more for less; doing more for a marginal increase in costs or doing more at no additional costs. Many hospitals have a cost improvement plan (CIP) based on efficiency [2].

P. Godbole
Department of Paediatric Surgery,
Sheffield Children's NHS Foundation Trust,
Sheffield, UK
e-mail: Prasad.Godbole@sch.nhs.uk

P. Godbole et al. (eds.), *Why Hospitals Fail*, DOI 10.1007/978-3-319-56224-7_16

The phenomenon of efficiency is obvious when one goes from the government sector to the private sector. In Government hospitals such as the National Health Service (U.K.) where all staff are salaried; there is very little incentive to be efficient as irrespective of outputs; salaries remain the same. It is only when the word 'transformation' or 'turnaround' is mentioned with resulting consequences such as workforce reviews that there is an incentive to be more efficient. Conversely, in a private hospital where the surgeon and his team are working on a performance related pay principle, the team works cohesively to get as many operations performed during the schedule.

As the definition of efficiency suggests, in hospitals this is predominantly to do with process [3]. Of course there may be slow surgeons and quicker surgeons as well as slower anaesthetists than others, but this is only part of the jigsaw and still remains within the process. Let us look at this process of a patient getting their operation and theatre scheduling in a bit more detail with the help of an example.

A secondary care hospital had significant problems with the number of patients being operated on a scheduled operating list. The process as outlined by the surgeons involved was that the theatre list was supposed to start at 9 am with knife to skin by the surgeon. However very rarely did this happen and more often than not the surgeon did not start till 0945. The interval between one patient being sent to the recovery room and the other patient being anaesthetised and brought into the OR was up to 45 min as there were delays in transporting the patients from their rooms to the OR and the scrub nurses not allowing the anaesthetist to start induction unless the instruments were checked. Furthermore patients were cancelled on the day due to being unwell or not adhering to preoperative starvation times/stopping their medications. Hence the total surgical time within the 4 h theatre schedule amounted to 30% i.e. of the 240 min available, the surgeon was only operating for (and generating income) for 80 min. This was clearly very inefficient as the fixed costs for running this operating schedule still had to be paid.

This would be a good opportunity to introduce the concept of LEAN management [4]. LEAN was a system used by the Toyota Production System that concentrated on eliminating or minimising processes that did not directly add value to the end product (processes in this setting = waste) and focusing on those that added value. The most significant effects on process value delivery are achieved by designing a process capable of delivering the required results smoothly. The Just in Time (JIT) philosophy of LEAN states "Make only what is needed, only when it is needed, and only in the amount that is needed".

How can this LEAN management system be implemented in our current example?

The main aim in our example was to have the right people in the right place at the right time with the right equipment to produce the desired result. If one were to remember this for the first patient and subsequent patients on the theatre schedule, the process improvement would be self evident. The process improvement (or efficiency) created was as follows:

1. It was mandated that the first patient on the list should be prepped and ready on the ward to arrive in the OR for 0845. It was left to individual wards and specialities to work backwards from this time to ensure that the patients arrived on time, were seen, checks done and patient prepped. The theatre orderlies/escorts/porters were called just in time to take the patient to the OR.
2. The theatre team had their preoperative brief at 0830
3. Theatre scheduling was done on a points system with every 15 min time slots awarded 1 point. Hence an operation that took a surgeon 30 min would be awarded 2 points. At the time of booking a patient on the theatre schedule the surgeon confirmed on the waiting list form the number of points needed for the surgery. The anaesthetist in the pre assessment (done on the same day) added the points for anaesthesia thereby allowing the full 4 h to be utilised.
4. The theatre list was signed off by the senior theatre manager 1 week before the list

5. The subsequent patient was sent for in time to arrive as the previous patient was handed over to recovery
6. The theatre scrub nurse checked the instruments as the patient was being anaesthetised (note any specific instrumentation would have been checked at the preoperative brief)
7. The operating surgeon had to be in theatre and scrubbed if appropriate when the patient was anaesthetised. Beware of the 'silent' surgeon sitting in the coffee room waiting to be called to the OR.

With the above process management; the surgical time increased to 60% and the theatre utilisation increased to over 90%.

So using the LEAN methodology what were the value laden aspects?

Work that is of direct value: Surgeon operating on a patient; this has to be maximised.

Work that contributes value: Patient needs to be asleep (anaesthetist).

Work that contributes value: Staff and equipment in a properly functioning OR.

Work that contributes value: Getting the patient to OR.

Work that contributes value: Ensuring patient arrives on time; has followed all instructions and is in good health.

LEAN management also encompasses continual process improvement [5]. Take the last element of work that contributes value in the above example.

The patient arriving on time: administrative process.

Has followed instructions: Pre assessment and administrative process.

Is in good health; how do we know?

Most patients may receive appointment letters, pre assessment letters about their surgery. However in this example, many patients either did not receive the letter of appointment and simply failed to turn up; had been ill a few days before and hence were cancelled or had not stopped their aspirin a week before. As part of the continual process improvement; a phone call was instituted 3–7 days before, asking three questions

1. Confirmation of the date of surgery and that nothing had changed in symptoms
2. Patient was aware of starving instructions and any other instructions given at the time of pre assessment
3. The patient's health had not changed

As can be seen by the above example, efficiency improved and throughput improved as a result.

However being efficient in itself is not a guarantee of success [6]. This will bring me on to the next part of effectiveness.

16.3 Effectiveness

Effectiveness is the capability of producing a desired result [7]. When something is deemed effective, it means it has an intended or expected outcome. If the same outcome can be expected and measured over and over again, this can be used as a quality measure.

There are four possible scenarios here:

1. A process may be efficient but ineffective
2. A process may be inefficient but effective
3. A process may be inefficient and ineffective
4. A process may be efficient and effective

	Effective	Ineffective
Efficient	4	1
Inefficient	2	3

Let us go back to our surgeons in the first example. Both are efficient and effective; the second more so than the first. Now if the first surgeon took another hour to do a sixth operation; this would increase staff and theatre costs; so although effective, it would be inefficient. If the second surgeon was efficient by doing six operations in the 4 hours, but two patients had complications needing further surgery; then he would be deemed efficient but ineffective. Finally if it took either surgeon significantly longer than the allocated 4 h AND had complications in two patients needing surgery; this would be inefficient and ineffective.

In many hospitals, management teams talk about cost effectiveness—but what exactly is it? This is nothing more than the amount in unit price it costs to achieve the desired result. So if we go back to our two surgeons; outcomes being equal for both; surgeon two would be more cost effective than surgeon one. Cost effectiveness has been used not only in hospitals but for allocation of healthcare resources [8] in many developed countries such as the U.K. In the U.K., anticancer drugs that cost thousands of dollars and prolong life for 3–6 months may be deemed not to be cost effective and therefore not provided on the NHS [9] and patients have to pay the costs for these drugs. This raises many ethical issues which is beyond the scope of this chapter.

In hospitals, similar cost effectiveness evaluations are used when considering new innovations and techniques. A simple example is the development of the minimally invasive laparoscopic techniques which superceded traditional (and in many cases historical) open techniques for surgery. Shorter hospital stay, quicker recovery and less pain, better cosmesis and the same outcomes made for this technique to be cost effective in appropriately trained hands. The invention of the Da Vinci Robot has taken minimally invasive surgery to the next level. But at a cost of $2 million would this be cost effective for a small secondary care hospital? Probably not.

As mentioned before effectiveness is about getting the expected and desired result every time. This has to be done in an efficient manner. This brings us to the next section on Six Sigma.

Six Sigma was introduced by Bill Smith in Motorola in 1986 [10]. The Six Sigma alludes to six standard deviations from the mean in terms of a defect free output. Or in other words, of all the outputs 99.99966% would have to be defect free. If Motorola were to make 1 million handsets then according to Six Sigma, no more than 3.4 could have defects. Hence Six Sigma is a process improvement set of tools for quality assurance purposes or ensuring quality outputs from given processes. While 99.99966% defect free may be aspirational in such processes; this does allow for continual process improvement.

Patients and their families are free to choose where they should have their treatment in most cases. Where a patient would like to go would depend on the condition to be treated; which hospital performs best in the treatment of the condition with best outcomes and experience of patients in the past. This shows the importance of efficiency and effectiveness. A hospital has to be efficient and effective to be adjudged a good hospital. In the U.K. patients are asked to give feedback by a friends and family test (FFT—[11]). This asks how likely the patient would be to recommend the hospital to their family and friends from a scale of very likely (best) to very unlikely (worst) with a free text box for comments. The best hospitals tend to have very high scores in their FFT (above 95–98%) with continual improvements in place to address any comments made.

We have considered the aspects of efficiency and effectiveness in hospitals. What happens when processes are lacking in both aspects? Chapter one demonstrated the downward spiral that a hospital can find itself in. It is in these circumstances that something has to change and transformation is part of the change process and will be discussed in the next section.

16.4 Types of Change

Change in healthcare is inevitable [12]. The chapters—What is change, Why do people resist change and overcoming change resistance give an in depth view of change management and the role of leadership within the change process.

Many management teams (mainly the not so experienced ones) describe changes they make as a transformation. So a change in the outpatient booking process would be coined outpatient transformation. This is incorrect and it is important to understand the various types of change with examples.

16.4.1 Development change

This is gradual and incremental and usual refines existing processes to improve what is currently being done [13]. So having extra chaperones on duty during busy outpatient clinic times would be a development change and not a transformation. Increasing or decreasing number of patients seen as agreed with the clinical staff—both for quality and safety and patient experience would be a developmental change.

16.4.2 Transitional change

In this change, the current state is replaced by a new state. Organisational changes to the way of working for various staff groups such as theatre staff, radiographers etc. would be a transitional change. The previous way of working needs to be replaced by the new way of working. There may be resistance but appropriate leadership and communication and engagement (standard change management tools) will allow this change to take place [14]). Transformational change is described below.

16.5 Transformational Change

This is probably the most drastic of all changes. For it to succeed it requires a complete change in mind set of everyone in the organisation; their behaviours; interpersonal relationships and turf wars [15]. The change is radical and although the organisation may have a umbrella change strategy and expected outcome; the implementation of the change may require constant manoeuvring and reassessing as the change progresses [16].

A great example of a transformational change in healthcare is the implementation of ObamaCare or The Affordable Care Act (ACA) in 2010. Under the act, hospitals and primary physicians would transform their practices financially, technologically, and clinically to drive better health outcomes, lower costs, and improve their methods of distribution and accessibility [17].

The Affordable Care Act was intended to increase health insurance quality and affordability, lower the uninsured rate by expanding insurance coverage and reduce the costs of healthcare. However this transformational change has led to a number of 'quality' measures the outcomes of which were hitherto unknown for hospital providers and hence would fit in with a transformational change. As a result of the ACA; a large number of previously uninsured people are insured and available to get treatment thereby increasing the hospital revenue. However in a bid to improve quality of healthcare; hospitals can be penalised and reimbursements withheld if patients return within 30 days of their discharge and are readmitted. Furthermore costs of healthcare previously uninsured such as breast pumps, screening for autism, aortic aneurysm screening are now included in the insurance thereby reducing the revenue. To avoid penalties; more of the treatment is being carried out in the outpatient setting which has a lower revenue. Incentives for electronic record keeping has led to several senior doctors retiring rather than spending money on the expensive electronic systems available. Since the election, hospitals are in limbo as to the future direction of this transformational change. At the time of going to print attempts to repeal the ACA has led to further uneasiness and anxiety due to uncertainty of the outcome.

Conclusion

Transformation, efficiency and effectiveness are the pillars of a successful hospital. They are linked to the finance, performance and quality and patient safety triad that every hospital has to juggle. LEAN and Six Sigma processes can be used to eliminate waste and for quality assurance purposes and continual improvement. Change can be varied with transformational change being the most radical, requiring a sea change in behaviours and mindset and strong leadership to make it successful.

Acknowledgements The author would like to acknowledge the contribution of the clinicians at the United Lincoln Hospital Trust for their collaboration and assistance work in the theatre utilisation project used as an example in this chapter.

References

1. ACHE. Top issues confronting hospitals in 2015. Available at https://www.ache.org/pubs/research/ceoissues/com.
2. Hurst J, Williams S. Can NHS hospitals do more with less? 2012. Available at www.nuffieldtrust.org/efficiency.
3. Harders M, Malangoni MA, Weight S, Sidhu T. Improving operating room efficiency through process redesign. Surgery. 2006;140(4):509–16.
4. Kim CS, Spahlinger DA, Kin JM, Billi JE. Lean health care: what can hospitals learn from a world class automaker? Soc Hosp Med. 2006;1(3):191–9.
5. Chen JC, Li Y, Shady BD. From value stream mapping toward a lean/sigma continuous improvement process: an industrial case study. Int J Prod Res. 2010;48(4):1069–86.
6. Takeuchi H, Osono E, Shimizu N. The contradictions that drive Toyota's success. Harv Bus Rev. 2008;96–105.
7. Drucker PF. The effective executive: the definitive guide to getting the right things done. New York: Collins; 2006.
8. Weinstein MC, Stason WB. Foundations of ciost-effectiveness analysis for health and medical practices. N Engl J Med. 1977;296:716–21.
9. Cancer Research UK. Health economics: the cancer drugs cost conundrum. 2016. Available at www.cancerresearchuk.org/funding-for-research.
10. Tennant G. Six sigma: SPC and TQM in manufacturing and services. Gower Publishing Ltd; 2001. p. 6.
11. NHS England. Friends and family test. 2014. Available at https://www.england.nhs.uk/ourwork/pe/fft/.
12. Choctaw WT. Change is inevitable. In: Choctaw WT, editor. A new paradigm for hospital and physician leadership in transforming the patient experience. Switzerland: Springer International Publishing; 2016. p. 1–2.
13. Marshak RJ. Managing the metaphors of change. Reflections. 1993;2:8.
14. Allen J, Jimmieson NL, Bordia P, Irmer BE. Uncertainty during organizational change: managing perceptions through communication. J Chang Manag. 2007;7(2):187–210.
15. Lukas CV, Holmes SK, Cohen AB, et al. Transformational change in healthcare systems: an organizational model. Healthcare Manage Rev. 2007;32(4):309–20.
16. Campbell RJ. Change management in healthcare. Health Care Manag. 2008;27(1):23–39.
17. Rosenbaum S. The patient protection and affordable care act: implications for public health policy and practice. Public Health Rep. 2011;126(1):130–5.

17 'Clinicians Versus Clinicians Versus Managers' or a New Patient Centred Culture That Eradicates 'Them and Us'?

Jill Aylott, Prasad Godbole, and Derek Burke

Doctors in the NHS are often singled out and blamed for individual behaviour that is sometimes labelled 'difficult' 'obstructive' 'resistant to change' and 'downright awkward'. In an English NHS system that is highly managed by a majority of non-clinicians at an NHS Trust Board level and controlled by politicians in terms of priorities and budget, an individual doctor's behaviour might better be understood within social identity theory (SIT) [1] as a normative response to an increasingly antagonistic context within the English NHS. SIT is a psychological theory that argues that a person's concept of 'self' comes from the groups to which the person belongs and that they will seek to identify with others who are also associated with this same group to help form a positive social identity, which will result in feelings of high esteem and positive wellbeing. Within hospitals, specialisms and sub-specialisms of medical and surgical practice creates highly skilled doctors and surgeons who work within increasingly highly specialised areas. Such a high level of specialism will require even closer attention to team working within health care to provide patients with a more holistic and patient centred service. However, in reality there might well be tensions between the objectives of team working and collective leadership and the motivation of individual specialists who seek to preserve their professional identity and the skills associated within their professional role. While clinicians seek to preserve their identity within their clinical role, they may not wish to participate in sharing medical/professional practice, which is suited both to their own skills and the skills of their colleagues, but will be defined separately within their own Royal Colleges' 'scope of practice'. This is a challenge for organisations who require more teamwork and sharing of practice, as services are transformed into new, more patient centred integrated care models.

This chapter will explore how doctors develop a positive Self Identity through their Royal Colleges 'scope of practice' and how the employing organisation or the wider context of healthcare practice seeks to challenge this scope of practice when disciplinary boundaries come under pressure as a result of staffing shortages in medicine, nursing and allied health professions [2]. Within this context there is very little self-determination [3–6] of doctors, (which is a

J. Aylott (✉)
Directorate for International MBA Programmes, International Academy of Medical Leadership, Sheffield, UK
e-mail: Jill.Aylott@iamedicalleadership.com

P. Godbole
Department of Paediatric Surgery, Sheffield Children's NHS Foundation Trust, Sheffield, UK
e-mail: Prasad.Godbole@sch.nhs.uk

D. Burke
Department of Emergency Medicine, Sheffield Children's NHS Foundation Trust, Sheffield, UK
e-mail: derek.burke@sch.nhs.uk

P. Godbole et al. (eds.), *Why Hospitals Fail*, DOI 10.1007/978-3-319-56224-7_17

critical condition for doctors to remain motivated and engaged), when the development of knowledge is constrained by a managerialist agenda [2, 7]. We will explore a specific case study of two medical specialities, Vascular Surgery and Interventional Radiology whose 'scope of practice' overlaps and argue for the introduction of (1) a quality improvement competency based programme for all clinicians and non-clinicians in healthcare and (2) the introduction of an organisational Quality Excellence award such as the European Foundation for Quality Excellence (EFQM). We argue that a QI competency framework combined with the EFQM could help to facilitate the development of team working across medical, clinical and non-clinical staff and focus all efforts to provide a high level of excellence in patient centred care. Such a focus on patient centred care will serve to focus the efforts of all team members emphasising an 'integrated model of care'.

Our case study will explore how Executive hospital leadership in the United States have developed new initiatives to 'integrate' surgical and radiology skills with a 'new' medical role in Vascular services. This project was successful in achieving an integrated social identity of vascular surgery and radiology which generated effective team working to deliver a quality service for patients. We go one step further and argue that to sustain collaborative working practices and to support effective team working, healthcare organisations should engage with the Quality Excellence model (EFQM), (Australian Quality Award or Baldrige Quality Award) which embeds the needs of its customers, patients and end users as being the primary focus for the business of healthcare, driving more demand for shared and overlapping multi-professional 'hybrid' roles.

We conclude with a recommendation that a healthcare organisation's leadership strategy should actively concern itself with the development of a patient centred quality improvement culture, that provides the rationale for the development of clinical and non-clinical competence. If such a step is not undertaken, then Social Identity Theory (SIT) explains that deep divisions will occur in the workforce and professionals will continue to become defensive and territorial about their own 'scope of practice'. The hospital executive board needs to act in a facilitative role to broker a more harmonious, happy and positive medical, clinical and non-clinical workforce.

Each of the Medical Royal Colleges or colleges of Nursing, physiotherapy and other professions in healthcare, are defined by a 'scope of practice' which sets out the legal and professional scope of practice of a given profession. Royal College specialties are further sub specialised. So for example the Royal College of Surgeons has separate register requirements for competence in general surgery and vascular surgery and the Royal College of Nursing is sub specialised to parts of the register for adult, child, mental health and learning disability nursing. A Scope of practice will inform 'credentialing' which is a verification of the experience and expertise of a scope of practice and also documents personal interest and willingness to provide medical or nursing care within this 'scope of practice'. This is used as a process to establish a contract between providers and commissioned work and is part of a process to award payment by private insurance companies for private healthcare. Credentialing is no longer just of interest or relevance to private insurance companies, but is increasingly relevant to doctors, nurses and the allied health professions working in healthcare who have to undergo revalidation every 3–5 years and who need to secure personal and professional indemnity insurance. While doctors currently go through a revalidation process it was a recommendation of the inquiry in the Mid Staffordshire hospital inquiry [8] that nurses will also have to undertake this process of professional revalidation in the UK in the future.

Social Identity Theory argues that the person's concept of self comes from the groups to which the person belongs. The person will have multiple selves and identities with their affiliated groups. There is also a psychological process of us aligning ourselves to the 'ingroup' and identifying the groups we don't belong to as the 'outgroups'. There are three processes that develop the in/out group thinking:

- Social categorisation—we categorise people in order to understand and identify them. In relation to the scope of practice of a professional group, we begin to know what categories we belong to and understand things about ourselves, defining and explaining appropriate behaviour according to the group we belong to. We can belong to several groups at the same time.
- Social Identification—we adopt the identity of the group that we belong to and act in ways that we understand and perceive we need to act in. In relation to the scope of practice of a profession, we develop an emotional significance to that identification and our self-esteem will depend on it.
- Social Comparison—After we have categorised ourselves within a group and identify ourselves as being members of that group, we tend to compare our group (the ingroup) against other groups (the outgroups). To maintain self-esteem we will compare our group favourably against other ones. A group will tend to view members of competing groups negatively to increase self-esteem.

SIT is always evidenced within a given context and with healthcare employing many different professional clinical roles and non-clinical roles, there will be significant opportunities to observe the effects of SIT. Studies have illustrated that extreme hostility can be induced by putting people into groups and then manipulating intergroup relations [9, 10]. Where groups exist in competition, where ones gain is the others loss—members will feel and act negatively towards each other. The theory calls against blaming individuals who respond to such arbitrary groupings and proposes that minimal conditions are necessary and sufficient to produce negativity towards outgroups. Studies have shown that the mere act of dividing people into groups can create antagonism. We define ourselves through the groups to which we belong. Social identities are much more than self perceptions: they also have value and emotional significance. To the extent that we define ourselves in terms of the group membership, our sense of self-esteem attaches to the fate of the group (and hence the fate of a fellow group members is pertinent to our own) [9]. The social nature of the bond is primary rather than secondary and we identify with others through our common link to a leader. This could explain how clinicians will feel a closer sense of connection to their Royal College with a secondary connection to the corporate values of the organisation We are bound together through our joint sense of belonging to the same category as our primary purpose.

17.1 Case Study: Vascular Surgeons and Interventional Radiologists

In the past, most vascular procedures were performed by Vascular Surgeons through large incisions that required hospitalisation with prolonged recuperation. Over the last few years advances in technology have seen the growth of endovascular procedures that are performed through a small tube placed in the artery. The removal of blockages in the artery or vein becomes a less invasive process for the patient and after the endovascular procedure, the patient recovers quickly and hospitalisation is unlikely to be required. The rapid development of endovascular techniques, while having a significant impact on both the diagnosis and treatment of patients with vascular disease, has at the same time also created conflict between the two main clinical specialists involved: interventional radiologists and vascular surgeons. The demand for endovascular techniques in the future will make up 40–70% [11] with possibly 90% in the future of vascular procedures being less invasive, as safer treatment modalities have evolved [11]. Scope of Practice will change and evolve over time, but registering changes or advances in 'scope of practice' services the legal and credentialing framework, it does not guarantee patients that a professional is a safe and competent practitioner. Canada has recognised that a Surgeon will change their scope of practice over time and provides guidance for this, however it also adds: "*the performance of innovative techniques or procedures within the context of a speciality or family of medicine, while new may not constitute a change of practice*".

It could be argued that the growth of endovascular surgery fits within this definition as it is the use of a particular technique that offers the Vascular Surgeon a wider range of skills to utilise in his/her intervention with patients. However, in 2010, in the UK, Consultant Radiologists developed a sub-specialty of radiology called 'interventional radiology' a new role created to provide this intervention within Vascular Services which had a major impact on both the professions of Vascular Surgeons and Radiologists. Although IR was officially given subspecialty status by the GMC in 2010—radiologists have been performing these procedures since these procedures were conceived by Charles Dotter and presented in his talk at the Czechoslovak Radiological Congress in 1963 [12]. While there are now attempts to understand the procedure as integrated 'Vascular Interventional Radiology' (VIR) the Royal Colleges continue to serve to represent the separate social identities of the separate medical professions of Radiologists and Vascular Surgeons.

Healthcare employing organisations have an important role to play in the facilitation of new and developed 'hybrid' roles that will deliver high quality of care to patients. The development of integrated service models, which are defined by clinical and non-clinical competencies will bring both vascular surgeons and interventional radiologists to the table to develop new service specifications of joint and collaborative team working. SIT could help to facilitate an understanding of the challenges and the tensions that could be encountered along the way. Working from a 'them' and 'us' position towards a people centred service for patients has been successful elsewhere [11, 13].

The lack of uniformity in credentialing criteria for the performance of endovascular procedures adds to the complexity of the problem and there have been calls to modify the training programmes most closely focused on vascular disease, vascular surgery and interventional radiology [11, 13]. The delivery of endovascular services differ substantially [11] and mini fellowships of 3 months in endovascular techniques are not seen as adequate for physicians with limited experience. It is recommended that any training programme solution must seek to 'up skill' all vascular surgeons to become proficient in endovascular techniques and for interventional radiologists to require broad clinical training in order to adequately and safely apply these new endovascular techniques. One such initiative is a 1 year integrated fellowship for interventionist radiologists and vascular surgeons where the evaluation found that the fellows support, like and recommend further integration of their roles. The fellowships were found to be mutually beneficial to both disciplines [11].

The case study of the emergence of endovascular procedures across two medical specialties scope of practice, highlights the tensions that can arise with the changing nature of medical practice with advances in technology and innovation. SIT illustrates the difficult and complex adjustment that is required of self-esteem of doctors in this fast changing healthcare context. What is considered by one Royal College as 'performance of innovative techniques or procedures within the context of a specialty or family of medicine (such as Vascular services) may be seen by another Royal College as a 'technique' or 'speciality' belonging to their own specialty's 'scope of practice'. In such situations employing organisations need to take a lead to develop integrated service models, where new skills are acquired by Vascular Surgeons and Interventional Radiologists and a team approach is facilitated. Only when this is achieved will the goal of offering high quality patient centred health procedures, within a team based culture, with less invasive procedures be delivered to patients.

The Quality Excellence Framework (EFQM Excellence Model) is a total quality framework [14] widely applied to healthcare in Italy [15] Holland [16] and Germany [17] with its American equivalent the Malcolm Baldrige award or the Australian Excellence award in Australia. The EFQM has nine dimensions which are grouped into five enablers and four results. The enablers describe how staff can improve: leadership, policy, strategy, people, partnerships and resources

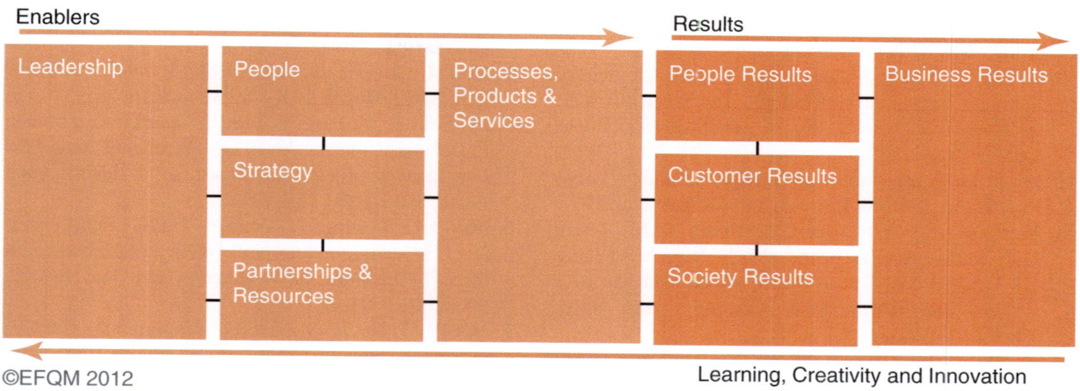

Fig. 17.1 The EFQM excellence model

and processes, while the results cover what the staff achieve: customer (patient feedback and satisfaction) people and society and key performance results. The model works primarily as a self-assessment tool which helps to prioritise improvements. The staff achieve a rating which is either a stage three, four or five level rating dependent on an external assessment and this process can support the integrated care model and support a competency approach with its balanced measures of processes and results (Fig.17.1).

The EFQM excellence model can stimulate greater accountability and support better performance results which ultimately improves patient quality in accessibility, safety, effectiveness, appropriateness and service efficiency [15]. With a UK shortage of Consultant Radiologists and 44% of NHS Trusts (93 out of 156) not offering interventional radiologists around the clock [18], the Excellence model could help provide a healthcare quality governance tool to identify specific action for upskilling and enabling a new hybrid role in endovascular services to achieve quality improvement. This would focus more effort into a new 'dual' hybrid role to meet the needs of patients instead of focusing on the development of uni-discipline specialties. As an improvement tool the Excellence model can connect and align healthcare governance and organisational structures and processes to increase quality across the healthcare system [15]. In an area such as endovascular services that is continuing to evolve across medical specialties, a more objective system wide improvement tool is required to keep a focus on the aspiration of excellence for patients.

Acknowledgements Dr. Rahil Kassamali interventional radiologist for his comments on earlier versions of this chapter.

References

1. Taifel H, Turner J. An intergrative theory of intergroup conflict. In: Austin WG, Worchel S, editors. The social psychology of intergroup relations. Monterey CA: Brooks/Cole; 1979. p. 33–48.
2. Nancarrow SA, Borthwick AM. Dynamic and professional boundaries in the healthcare workforce. Sociol Health Illn. 2005;29(7):897–919.
3. Deci RL, Ryan RM. Intrinsic motivation and self-determination in human behaviour. New York: Plenum Press; 1985.
4. Deci EL, Ryan RM. The 'what' and 'why' of goal pursuits: human needs and the self determination of behaviour. Psychol Inq. 2000;11(4):227–68.
5. Deci EL, Vansteenkiste M. Self-determination theory and basic need satisfaction: understanding human development in positive psychology. Ricerchedi Psichologia. 2004;27:17–34.
6. Ryan RM, Deci EL. Self-determination theory and the facilitation of intrinsic motivation, social development and well-being. Am Psychol. 2000;55(1):68–78.
7. Martin G. Interprofessional boundaries. In: Cockerham W, Dingwall R, Quah S, editors. The Wiley Blackwell encyclopedia of health and illness, behaviour and society. London: Wiley; 2014.

8. Francis R. The report into the inquiry of mid staffordshire hospital. 2013.
9. Reicher S, Spears S, Haslam SA. The social identity approach in social psychology. In: Wetherall MS, Mohanty CT, editors. Social identities handbook. London: Sage; 2010.
10. Sherif M. Group conflict and co-operation: their social psychology. London: Routledge and Kegan Paul; 1967.
11. Messina LM, Schneider DB, Chuter TAM, Reilly LM, Kerlan RK, LaBerge JM, Wilson MW, Ring EJ, Gordon RL. Integrated fellowship in vascular surgery and intervention radiology. Ann Surg. 2002;236(4):408–15.
12. Rosch J, Keller FS, Kaufman JA. The birth, early years and future of interventional radiology. J Vasc Interv Radiol. 2003;14:841–53.
13. Green RM, Waldman DL. Five year results of a merger between vascular surgeons and interventional radiologists in a university medical center: implications for training. J Vasc Inter Radiol. 2003;38(6):1213–7.
14. EFQM. Introducing the EFQM model: EFQM Excellence Model. 2010. www.efqm.org
15. Favaretti C, De Pieiri P, Torri E, Guarrera G, Fontana F, Debiasi F, Flor L. An EFQM excellence model for integrated healthcare govrnance. Int J Healthc Qual Assur. 2015;28(2):156–72.
16. Nabitz U, Klazinga N, Walburg J. The EFQM excellence model: European and Dutch experiences with the EFQM approach in healthcare. Int J Qual Healthc. 2000;12(3):191–201.
17. Moeller J. The EFQM excellence model: the German experience with the EFQM approach in healthcare. Int J Healthc. 2001;13(1):45–9.
18. The Royal College of Radiologists and the British Society of Interventional Radiology. Investing in the interventional radiology workforce: the quality and efficiency case. 2014.

Index

P. Godbole et al. (eds.), *Why Hospitals Fail*, DOI 10.1007/978-3-319-56224-7

MIX
Papier aus verantwortungsvollen Quellen
Paper from responsible sources
FSC® C105338

If you have any concerns about our products,
you can contact us on
ProductSafety@springernature.com

In case Publisher is established outside the EU,
the EU authorized representative is:
Springer Nature Customer Service Center GmbH
Europaplatz 3, 69115 Heidelberg, Germany

Printed by Libri Plureos GmbH
in Hamburg, Germany